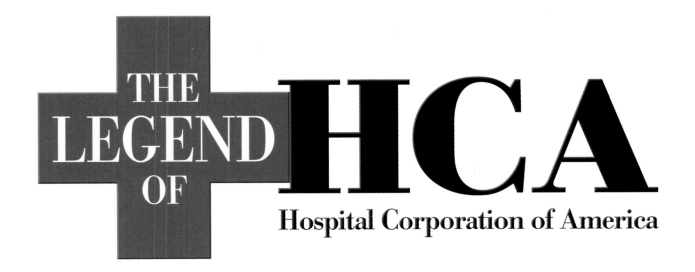

THE LEGEND OF HCA

Hospital Corporation of America

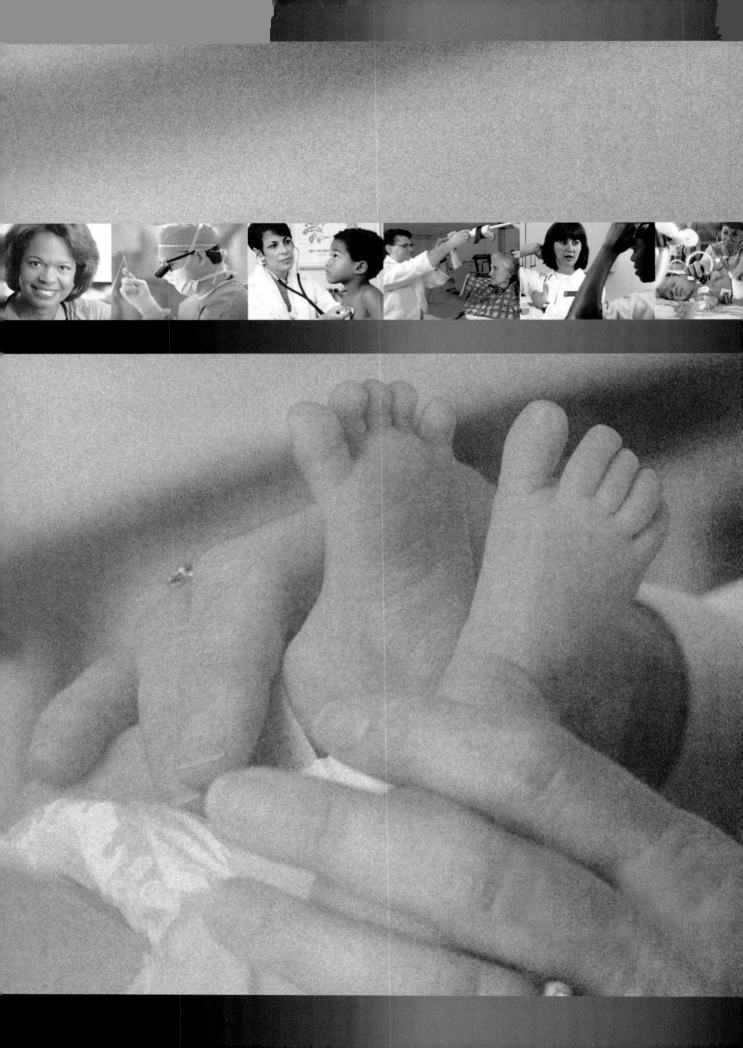

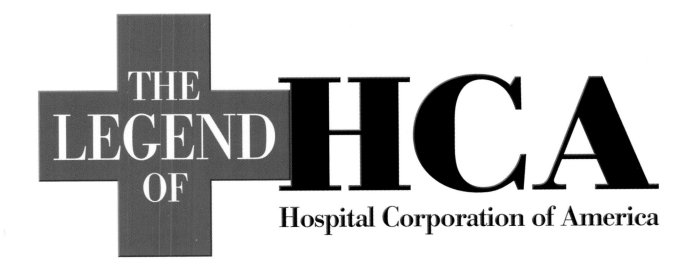

THE LEGEND OF HCA

Hospital Corporation of America

JEFFREY L. RODENGEN

Edited by Melody Maysonet
Design and layout by Sandy Cruz and Rachelle Donley

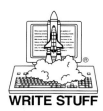

WRITE STUFF

Write Stuff Enterprises, Inc.
1001 South Andrews Avenue
Second Floor
Fort Lauderdale, FL 33316
1-800-900-Book (1-800-900-2665)
(954) 462-6657
www.writestuffbooks.com

Publisher's Cataloging-in-Publication

Rodengen, Jeffrey L.
    The legend of HCA / Jeffrey L. Rodengen ; edited by Melody Maysonet ; design and layout by Sandy Cruz and Rachelle Donley. -- 1st ed.
    p. cm.
    Includes bibliographical references and index.
    ISBN 0-945903-83-9

    1. HCA (Firm)--History. 2. Medical corporations--United States   I. Title.

    R728.2.R634 2003   362.1'1
                        QBI03-200657

Library of Congress
Catalog Card Number 2001131633

ISBN 0-945903-83-9

Completely produced in the
United States of America
10 9 8 7 6 5 4 3 2 1

Also by Jeff Rodengen

The Legend of Chris-Craft

IRON FIST: The Lives of Carl Kiekhaefer

Evinrude-Johnson and The Legend of OMC

Serving the Silent Service: The Legend of Electric Boat

The Legend of Dr Pepper/Seven-Up

The Legend of Honeywell

The Legend of Briggs & Stratton

The Legend of Ingersoll-Rand

The Legend of Stanley: 150 Years of The Stanley Works

The MicroAge Way

The Legend of Halliburton

The Legend of York International

The Legend of Nucor Corporation

The Legend of Goodyear: The First 100 Years

The Legend of AMP

The Legend of Cessna

The Legend of VF Corporation

The Spirit of AMD

The Legend of Rowan

New Horizons: The Story of Ashland Inc.

The History of American Standard

The Legend of Mercury Marine

The Legend of Federal-Mogul

Against the Odds: Inter-Tel—The First 30 Years

The Legend of Pfizer

State of the Heart: The Practical Guide to Your Heart and Heart Surgery
with Larry W. Stephenson, M.D.

The Legend of Worthington Industries

The Legend of IBP, Inc.

The Legend of Trinity Industries, Inc.

The Legend of Cornelius Vanderbilt Whitney

The Legend of Amdahl

The Legend of Litton Industries

The Legend of Gulfstream

The Legend of Bertram
with David A. Patten

The Legend of Ritchie Bros. Auctioneers

The Legend of ALLTEL
with David A. Patten

The Yes, you can of Invacare Corporation
with Anthony L. Wall

The Ship in the Balloon: The Story of Boston Scientific and the Development of Less-Invasive Medicine

The Legend of Day & Zimmermann

The Legend of Noble Drilling

Fifty Years of Innovation: Kulicke & Soffa

Biomet—From Warsaw to the World
with Richard F. Hubbard

NRA: An American Legend

The Heritage and Values of RPM, Inc.

The Marmon Group: The First Fifty Years

The Legend of Grainger

The Legend of The Titan Corporation
with Richard F. Hubbard

The Legend of Discount Tire Co.
with Richard F. Hubbard

The Legend of Polaris
with Richard F. Hubbard

The Legend of La-Z-Boy
with Richard F. Hubbard

The Legend of McCarthy
with Richard F. Hubbard

InterVoice: Twenty Years of Innovation
with Richard F. Hubbard

Jefferson-Pilot Financial: A Century of Excellence
with Richard F. Hubbard

TABLE OF CONTENTS

INTRODUCTION

WHEN DR. THOMAS FRIST SR., his son Dr. Thomas Frist Jr., and Jack Carroll Massey founded Hospital Corporation of America (HCA) in 1968, they started a revolution in the healthcare industry, not only in Nashville, where the company began, but across the entire country. HCA was one of the first investor-owned hospital companies in the nation. As such, the company pioneered an entirely new way of running hospitals. The three founders combined their experience and abilities to achieve the highest standards of patient care while attaining significant cost savings in the architecture, construction, and management of hospitals. To combat the rapidly spiraling cost of healthcare, HCA applied management techniques from other industries, streamlined operations and purchasing, and eliminated waste and inefficiencies. As Jack Massey observed in 1969, "We believe that a corporate chain of hospitals, using private capital, with physicians involved in management, can provide superior healthcare while solving many of the problems confronting the hospital industry."

Massey was correct, but neither he nor the Drs. Frist suspected they were making history when they purchased Park View Hospital in 1968 and set about building and acquiring a network of hospitals.

The overarching goal of the founders was to improve patient care. According to Dr. Frist Sr., HCA was created to fulfill "a community need for superior hospital care at the lowest possible cost." Frist Sr. promised that "HCA management [was] dedicated, above all, to warmth and compassion for the patients in its hospitals." The founders resolved that they would not build, acquire, or manage hospitals unless they met certain high standards, and all would be run according to Dr. Frist Sr.'s humanitarian philosophy.

Despite the founders' altruistic philosophy, critics accused companies like HCA of being in business only to make a profit. On the contrary, HCA reinvested its profit in its people, facilities, and technology, all toward the goal of delivering superior healthcare. It became intimately involved in communities, brought jobs, and paid federal, state, and local taxes. Moreover, HCA's ability to raise capital to build hospitals filled a serious need, for HCA hospitals provided first-class facilities and equipment that attracted new doctors.

Over the years, HCA has been a leader in balancing and improving the nation's healthcare system. In 1985, after the federal government froze Medicare payments to hospitals, HCA was the first investor-owned hospital company to announce that its earnings would be affected, an openness later appreciated by investors. Dr. Frist Jr. and HCA's other leaders began "right-sizing," an effort other hospital companies soon imitated. Later, HCA recognized that the Balanced Budget Act of 1997 was cutting Medicare reimbursements much deeper than Congress intended. The company helped initiate a grassroots campaign to correct the matter. Ultimately, Congress passed the Balanced Budget Refinement Act, which reduced future Medicare cuts, and the Benefit Improvement and Protection Act, which helped compensate for the extensive reductions. When HCA realized it wasn't getting a fair return from its managed care contracts, it renegotiated them, prompting other hospitals to do the same. HCA was the first hospital company to set up an infrastructure for sharing administrative and business services among its hospitals, and it was the first to create a formal program to improve patient safety by reducing the number of medical errors. But perhaps HCA's greatest contribution has been to serve as a stimulus for changing the predominantly not-for-profit cottage industry into an organized and efficient system for hospital management.

HCA's influence on healthcare is especially acute in Nashville, where a series of acquisitions, mergers, and spin-offs involving HCA and its seasoned executives soon made the Tennessee capital the epicenter of the investor-owned healthcare industry. Known in some circles as the Silicon Valley of Healthcare, Nashville is home to more than 450 healthcare companies and industry support firms, many of which sprang from HCA or Nashville-based Hospital Affiliates International (HAI), which HCA acquired in 1981. Dr. Frist Jr., Jack Bovender Jr. (current HCA chairman and CEO), and former HCA leaders played a key role in establishing the Nashville Health Care Council (NHCC), an association of healthcare leaders created to foster Nashville's healthcare industry. According to the NHCC, "The founding of HCA created a spark in Nashville's business community that helped the area build an empire of healthcare management and related companies in little more than three decades."

In the 1970s and early 1980s, HCA went through a number of incarnations as the healthcare industry evolved. A rapid series of acquisitions coupled with a rush of new construction and hospital management contracts soon made HCA a billion-dollar company comprising 350 hospitals. In the early 1980s, HCA diversified into other healthcare ventures when antitrust concerns raised questions about future growth through hospital acquisitions, only to move back to its roots and undergo massive restructuring after the Medicare amendments of 1983 and the rapid rise of HMOs shocked hospitals into drastic cost cutting. In 1988, when public hospital stocks were undervalued and corporate takeovers by leveraged buyout (LBO) firms were in vogue, Dr. Frist Jr. and an HCA management group took the company private in an LBO. HCA spent three years as a private company, repaying loans and selling off noncore assets. When it went public again in 1992, it enjoyed a smaller and stronger core group of assets, a focused strategy, and renewed access to equity capital.

In the early 1990s, as the country's healthcare system became mired in the managed care revolution, Frist Jr. made the difficult decision to merge with Columbia Hospital Corporation (a smaller company with a higher price-earnings multiple) in order to grow. The old adage "Be careful what you wish for" certainly applied. The merger was completed in February 1994, and for the next three years, Columbia/HCA grew at an astounding rate. But the growth came too fast. Without adequate infrastructure enhancements, numerous nonhospital businesses were bought, and individual hospitals began to suffer. Dr. Frist Jr. watched helplessly in his new role as vice chairman as the company he helped create seemed to come apart at the seams. This passage reached its climax when the Department of Justice began probing Columbia's operations in early 1997.

After Columbia chairman and CEO Rick Scott resigned, Dr. Frist Jr. stepped back into the role of company leader, and Jack Bovender rejoined as president and chief operating officer. The two friends worked to resolve the investigations, mend the company's reputation, and strengthen HCA's commitment to the care and improvement of human life. Columbia/HCA became, once again, HCA, or to many, Hospital Corporation of America.

HCA's renaissance involved paring down the number of hospitals it operated, returning to a community focus, and strengthening operations. But perhaps most important, it involved renewing the values on which it was founded, values based on bringing the best possible care to patients, respecting the dignity of the individual, and recognizing that its greatest asset is its people.

When he was 87 years old, Dr. Thomas Frist Sr. wrote a letter to his future great-grandchildren. The letter, penned less than a month before he died, demonstrates his wisdom and reinforces his legacy and that of the company he helped create. "I believe good people beget good people," he wrote. "That's how we built Hospital Corporation of America.... We wanted good people with integrity and high moral standards. We made such a difference in the world with HCA, and we did it because good people beget good people."

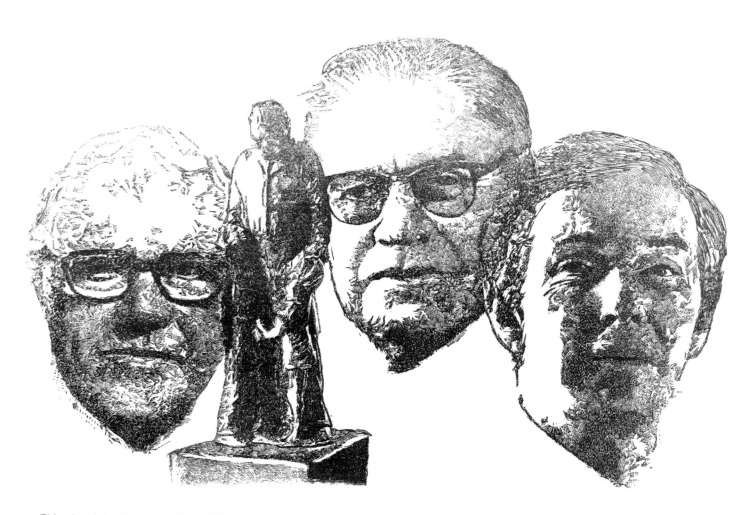

This sketch by Dan Quist titled "The Spirit of HCA" depicts HCA founders (from left) Jack Massey, Dr. Thomas Frist Sr., and Dr. Thomas Frist Jr., along with a statue of Dr. Frist Sr. with his arms around two children. The original bronze statue, known as the Dr. Thomas F. Frist Sr. Humanitarian Award, is a symbol of the company's dedication to quality patient care. The statue is awarded each year to an HCA employee and a volunteer who show particular compassion for patients.

ACKNOWLEDGMENTS

MANY PEOPLE ASSISTED IN THE research, preparation, and publication of *The Legend of HCA.*

This book would not have been possible without the professional skills of our talented research assistants, James Summerville and Candace Floyd. James's writing and research talents went a long way toward making this book a success, and Candace's diligence in finding hard-to-locate photos is much appreciated. Melody Maysonet, senior editor, oversaw the text and photos from beginning to end, and graphic design by Rachelle Donley and Sandy Cruz brought the story to vivid life.

Several key people associated with HCA lent their invaluable efforts to the book's completion, sharing their experience, providing valuable oversight for accuracy, and helping guide the book's development from outline to final form: Dr. Thomas Frist Jr., Victor Campbell, and Jeff Prescott. In addition, Terri Hicks was a great help in coordinating communication, and Laura Campbell reviewed early manuscript drafts.

Many other HCA executives, employees, retirees, and friends greatly enriched the book by discussing their experiences. The author extends particular gratitude to these men and women for their candid recollections: David Anderson, Peter Bird, Jack Bovender, Richard Bracken, Helen King Cummings, Rosalyn Elton, Jim Fitzgerald, Carl George, Sam Hazen, John Hindelong, Dr. Frank Houser, Milton Johnson, Trish Lindler, Steve Riven, Bill Rutherford, Joe Steakley, Bob Waterman, Noel Williams, and Alan Yuspeh.

Special thanks are extended to the dedicated staff and associates at Write Stuff Enterprises, Inc.: Richard Hubbard, executive author; Jon VanZile, executive editor; Heather Deeley, associate editor; Bonnie Freeman, copyeditor; Dennis Shockley, art director; Mary Aaron, transcriptionist; Barbara Koch, indexer; Bruce Borich, production manager; Marianne Roberts, vice president of administration; Sherry Hasso, bookkeeper; Linda Edell, executive assistant to Jeffrey L. Rodengen; Lars Jessen, director of worldwide marketing; Irena Xanthos, manager of sales, promotions, and advertising; and Rory Schmer, distribution supervisor.

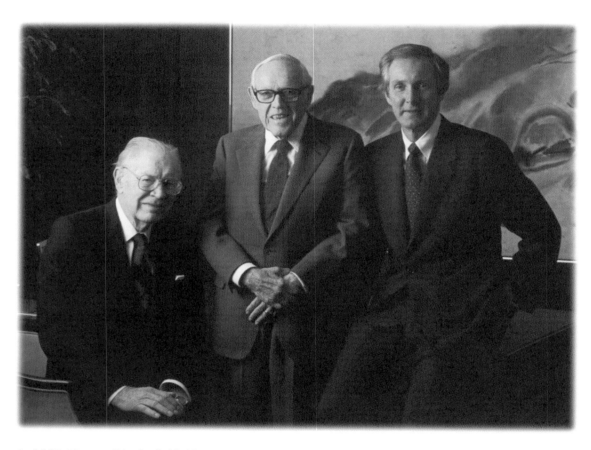

In 1968, Thomas Frist Sr. (left), his son Thomas Frist Jr. (right), and Jack Massey (center) joined forces to found Hospital Corporation of America.

CHAPTER ONE

GREAT MINDS CONVERGE

1968–1969

Bettering the human condition is the greatest good any individual can achieve.

—Dr. Thomas Frist Sr.

TWENTY-EIGHT-YEAR-OLD DR. Thomas Frist Jr., one of Hospital Corporation of America's cofounders, spent much of the tumultuous decade of the 1960s earning his premed degree at Vanderbilt University and his M.D. at Washington University School of Medicine. Afterwards, he returned to Nashville for his surgical internship and residency.[1]

But in common with many of his generation, Tommy Frist Jr. had his surgical residency interrupted when he was called into the United States Air Force during the Vietnam War. He was assigned to duty as a flight surgeon at the Warner Robins Air Force Base outside Macon, Georgia, where he had time to reflect upon something his father had told him years before. "Medicine opens up so many avenues for you. You can be a great general practitioner, a great specialist. You can do research, be in government, or use your medical degree as a lawyer, entrepreneur, or businessman—just so many things."[2]

The profession seemed to run in his family. His two brothers would become successful heart surgeons, and his father was a doctor.

"My father never told me what to do, or not to do," Frist Jr. related. Regardless, he had an uneasy moment when he picked up the telephone to tell his dad, a prominent, well-respected cardiologist, that he didn't want to practice medicine after all. Instead he wanted to be one of the founders of a yet-to-be-named hospital company.[3]

Modest Beginnings

Dr. Thomas Fearn Frist Sr., Tommy's father, had found his vocation early in life.

Born in Meridian, Mississippi, in 1910, the boy was eight years old when his father, Jacob Chester Frist, was fatally struck by a train after saving a woman and her baby from the railroad tracks where he worked as a station master. Frist Sr.'s mother became the family breadwinner, supporting her two sons and two daughters by running a boarding house that catered to teachers and doctors.[4]

"Among our guests were a physician and a minister," Dr. Frist Sr. once recollected. "I had the experience of sitting down and talking with them at the dinner table. I guess they became role models for my brother and me [because my brother] became a Presbyterian minister."[5]

In 1923 the youngster took a job in a hospital to help his mother make ends meet. "I grew to love hospitals," Frist Sr. said. "I never had any thought other than being a doctor. It is the most rewarding thing a person can possibly be in life."

This corporate logo appeared in HCA's 1969 annual report, which informed shareholders that the company "now serves 24 communities in seven states with 26 high-quality hospitals offering superior patient care to the people of those areas."

The lad worked his way through the University of Mississippi, taking various jobs such as picking up and delivering laundry, selling white coats to medical students, and calling play-by-play action at football games. He also met his fellow students arriving by train and hauled their trunks with a mule and a dray. He soon learned a little something about business competition when others started offering the same service. So young Frist Sr. began traveling up the line, meeting students on the way into Oxford and getting their orders in advance. When his various moneymaking endeavors proved too difficult for one person to handle, he hired other students. By the time he graduated from the university, he had 17 people working for him.[6]

In 1931 Thomas Frist Sr., 18 years old and nearly penniless, arrived at Vanderbilt University School of Medicine in Nashville to begin medical school. But recalling his mother's successful enterprise, he persuaded Mrs. Jennie Compton, a widow, to allow him to act as agent for a boarding house that she owned in Nashville within a short walk of Vanderbilt's hospital. "I wrote all the students in medical school and asked them if they wanted to live in 'Pauper's Paradise,'" Frist Sr. remembered. "They got a room and two meals a day for $15 a month. I got room and board free."[7]

The young man had the opportunity to study with some of the most illustrious names in the history of Vanderbilt, men such as Sidney Burwell, Hugh Morgan, Tinsley Harrison, and John Youmans. They belonged to the first generation of faculty in the "new" medical school, recently rebuilt and reformed along scientific lines with Rockefeller money. Frist Sr. listened as Dr. Harrison taught his young charges about the workings of the heart by mimicking its sounds: the lub-dub of the valves accentuated by screeches and whistles. Frist Sr. took special interest in internal medicine and in cardiology. He served his internship at the University of Iowa Hospital, then returned to Nashville in 1935 and entered private practice.[8] He specialized in cardiology and became an active member of the Nashville Academy of Medicine and of the Southeastern Clinical Club.[9]

During World War II, Frist Sr. reported to active military duty in Montgomery, Alabama, in the U.S. Army Medical Corps, where he became chief of medical services for a 1,000-bed hospital.

He was discharged as a major at war's end and returned to Nashville. After a few years at his downtown headquarters, he moved his practice to a converted West End Avenue mansion, which he purchased at cost from friend Jack Massey, who years later would also become one of HCA's cofounders. Frist Sr. had met Massey shortly after Frist entered private practice in 1935.

Frist Sr. was quite active in the medical profession and in community work. In 1949 he represented Vanderbilt University as a member of the City of Nashville and Davidson County Hospital Authority. In 1950 he became cochairman of the Middle Tennessee Heart Association's fundraising activities. In 1958 he began serving as president-elect of Saint Thomas Hospital and joined Nashville General Hospital's board of commissioners.[10]

In 1957, Dr. Frist Sr. was appointed to the American Medical Association (AMA) Committee on Aging. "All of a sudden, we found ourselves with about 11 million people over 65 [and] no one thinking about their future," Frist Sr. said. "This was before Medicare and all the other programs we now take for granted about care for the aging." Frist Sr. subsequently established the Tennessee Commission on Aging, which was financed by the state.[11]

"At that time there were no decent nursing homes in Nashville, not a single one, nor were there any private homes for the elderly," Frist Sr. recalled. At an AMA Committee on Aging meeting, Frist Sr. said he "was going to come back in two years and show them the finest nursing home combined with a hospital anywhere in the world." Frist Sr. kept that promise. It was called Park View Convalescent Hospital and Nursing Home.[12]

Park View Hospital

Dr. Frist Sr.'s early love of hospitals never left him, but as a practicing physician he often became frustrated when he wanted to admit a patient to a Nashville institution. Though he was on the faculty of Vanderbilt's medical school, he could not get his patients into its hospital without lengthy delay. It was no help that he served on the executive committee of Saint Thomas Hospital, a voluntary hospital, and on the board of the city's general hospital; they too had no room.[13]

"I was very much concerned with the quality of the medical care people were getting," Frist Sr. recalled, "particularly the lack of warmth and compassion and kindness and friendliness to the patient and his family. The other hospitals were so crowded and so independent that they had, to a large degree, lost the humanitarian aspect of medicine which I think is so important for the happiness and welfare of the patient."[14]

A privately owned hospital would not be dependent on government funds or donations but would operate in the private enterprise system, pay taxes, and run on a businesslike program, all while rendering a great service.[15]

In 1960 Frist Sr.'s experiences with hospitals led him, along with 20 medical colleagues and four Nashville businessmen, to begin building a place for patients on a site near Nashville's famed replica of the Parthenon in Centennial Park. Each investor in the partnership put up $11,000 of his own money; then collectively the group borrowed $1.2 million from the National Life and Accident Insurance Company.[16]

For the hospital he recruited top-notch personnel: "the best housekeeper, the best director of nursing, the best dietician, the best x-ray man. All of them stayed for more than 20 years," Frist Sr. said. "And we formed a cohesive group between doctors and the board, all working in concert." Rooms were painted in pastel colors. Halls had paintings and sculptures, and lounges offered comfortable chairs in front of television sets. A glass-enclosed solarium and sun deck topped the fourth floor.[17]

Park Vista Convalescent Hospital and Nursing Home opened in December 1961 with 152 beds for the care of patients no longer in the critical stage of illness but still in need of care. Costs ranged from $9 a day upward, compared to an average of $25 at a general hospital. The name later changed to Park View Hospital.[18]

"The less sick you are, the less you pay," noted Dr. Frist Sr., who added that such an operating concept worked "extremely well."[19]

Park View grew. In 1965 the owners recruited other physicians and added a $1.5 million surgical wing, converting Park View, now with 200 beds, from a strictly convalescent facility.[20] "Our hospital prospered so well because of the warmth

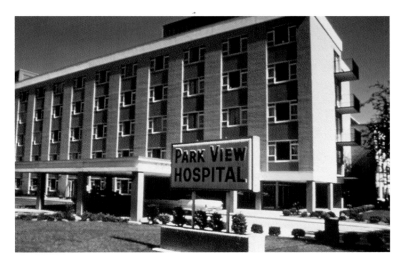

Park View Hospital was established in Nashville in 1961 by Thomas Frist Sr. and other Nashville doctors, who contributed $11,000 each and borrowed $1.2 million from Nashville-based National Life and Accident Insurance Company. In June 1968, the newly formed Hospital Corporation of America acquired Park View from its physician-owners through an offering of stock valued at $5 million.

and compassion and kindness," said Frist Sr. "Doctors [also] liked it because of the good food and its neat, clean appearance."[21]

By 1967, Park View had become so successful that its owners, now totaling 62, could not come up with enough private capital to meet their growing needs. This same story—a small institution backed with private capital facing new, costly demands for more space, more equipment, and more services— was echoing throughout the country, especially in the Sun Belt states.

Dr. Frist Sr. and the attorney for Park View, Henry Hooker, came up with a plan to deed Park View to the city. They proposed that a special not-for-profit general welfare corporation called Westside Public Hospital Corporation buy the hospital using tax-exempt bonds, hold it until revenues had paid off the debt, then deed it to the metropolitan government. Mayor Beverly Briley at first expressed interest.[22] Nashville owned and operated a general hospital built around a 19th-century physical plant that was in dire need of improvement. Dr. Frist Sr.'s facility was, by comparison, relatively new.

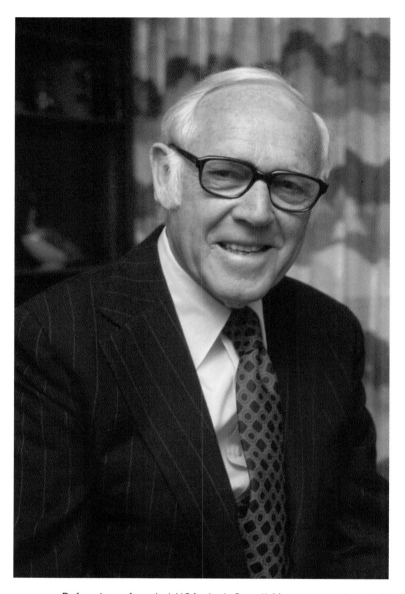

Before he cofounded HCA, Jack Carroll Massey owned a retail drugstore, founded a surgical supply company, and was one of the builders of Baptist Hospital in Nashville. He also bought Kentucky Fried Chicken for $2 million in 1964, selling the chain in 1971 for common stock valued at about $239 million.

But instead of passing to public ownership, a year later Park View would become the flagship institution for a new company—Hospital Corporation of America (HCA)—and a vast new American industry.

"Business Is People"

Jack Carroll Massey, HCA's third cofounder, was the legendary business genius who had made Kentucky Fried Chicken the spectacular success it was. Trained as a pharmacist, Massey had owned a retail drugstore, founded a successful Nashville surgical supply company, and owned or had interests in a half-dozen other businesses. He was also among the leaders of Baptist Hospital, one of Nashville's largest and most popular voluntary hospitals, and served as its president for a dozen years. Over the years, he proved his business savvy by raising $1 million to improve Baptist Hospital and another $2.5 million to expand it. He, like Frist Sr., was active in the community.[23]

Frist Sr. recalled that during the Great Depression, Massey Surgical Supply sold supplies to many hospitals that were unable to pay for them. Rather than cutting the hospitals off, "Mr. Massey established a team to help the people operate the hospital in a businesslike, efficient way."[24]

After opening Massey Surgical Supply Company's fourth facility, Massey sold the firm in 1961 to take early retirement in Florida. The 56-year-old entrepreneur soon found leisure life a bore and set out to find a new challenge. In 1964 he and a young attorney named John Y. Brown, who later became governor of Kentucky, bought Kentucky Fried Chicken from "Colonel" Harlan Sanders. The new owners guaranteed the colorful Colonel a $40,000 annual salary for life to promote the restaurants. In exchange, they received full rights to all patents and trademarks.[25]

As principal shareholder, chairman, and chief executive officer, Massey went to work to boost the fortunes of Kentucky Fried Chicken. His primary focus was human resources. "Business is people," Massey once observed. "People are our most important asset."[26] This was a philosophy he would carry over to HCA.

There followed a seven-year period of astonishing growth. Kentucky Fried Chicken was not merely one of the first fast-food chains; it reached the pinnacle of the fast-food-chain industry and ultimately became the most successful chain in the industry.

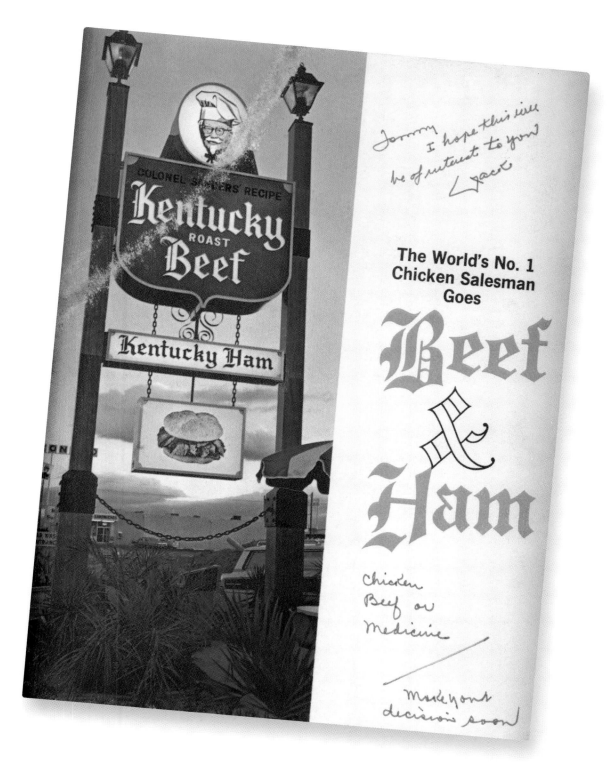

As Frist Jr. pondered his future, Kentucky Fried Chicken chairman and CEO Jack Massey prodded him to decide quickly. "Chicken, beef or medicine. Make your decision soon," Massey wrote to the young Frist Jr.

When KFC was listed on the New York Stock Exchange (NYSE) in 1969, it became one of three companies Massey would take to the Big Board. He was the first person in NYSE history to accomplish such a feat.

Memphis or Nashville?

Meanwhile, the road map for what would become Hospital Corporation of America began to take shape. Whiling away the time between patients in the sick bay at Warner Robins Air Force Base, Tommy Frist Jr. had observed the impact Jack Massey had made at KFC through applying basic business principles to a "mom and pop" company. He saw the same evolutionary process occurring in other sectors of the economy, such as consolidation of grocery stores, banks, and hotels. And, in fact, it was the "up close" experience of watching Kemmons Wilson (the father of his Vanderbilt fraternity brother Spence Wilson), who founded Holiday Inn of America in Memphis, that provided the catalyst for Dr. Frist Jr. to approach his father about creating a publicly owned multi-hospital company.[27]

In the 1950s, Kemmons Wilson and fellow Holiday Inn of America founder Wallace Johnson had revolutionized the travel and leisure industry with the creation of Holiday Inn. In the mid-1960s, using many of the same concepts, Wilson and Johnson founded a nursing home company called Medicenters of America.

Recognizing that 5,000-plus hospitals throughout the United States were being run as a cottage industry, Dr. Frist Jr. wondered if hospitals could be linked like chain motels. In 1967 David Jones and Wendell Cherry founded and took public a nursing home chain called Extendicare, which gave further credibility to Dr. Frist Jr.'s concept. These were the go-go years in the stock market, and the overnight doubling of the IPOs of Medicenters and Extendicare did not go unnoticed by the entrepreneurially oriented young surgeon. He suggested to his father that Dr. Frist Sr. approach Kemmons Wilson about merging Park View Hospital with Medicenters, whose shares he owned. Park View Hospital's earnings of $400,000 exceeded all the earnings of the 14 Medicenters nursing homes.[28]

The proposal was not well received, however. "They thought that the nursing home was the right answer," said Frist Jr., "and they still had the general feeling that there was no money to be made in hospital management."[29] Meanwhile, the 1967 proposal that the hospital be deeded to the city had gone nowhere.

"Let's Do It"

Frist Jr. proposed to Massey and his father that they join the three hospitals in which Frist Sr. was involved. By that time, Frist Sr. had built Park View, helped build a badly needed 52-bed hospital in Lewisburg, Tennessee (Taylor Hospital), and was involved in planning a new hospital to replace the ailing Donelson Hospital in suburban Nashville.[30]

In February 1968, Tommy Frist Jr. got word from his dad that Frist Sr., Henry Hooker, and Jack Massey were meeting the next Sunday morning to discuss Massey's proposal to buy a Nashville bank. "Dad mentioned that it might be possible to interject the idea of forming a company at the meeting to own all three hospitals in which he was an investor," Frist Jr. recalled.[31]

That next Sunday, Massey, Hooker, and the Drs. Frist met and drew up plans for a hospital company that, in the words of Dr. Frist Sr., would fulfill "a community need for superior hospital care at the lowest possible cost" and that would prove profitable to its investors. It would own, not franchise, and it would acquire existing hospitals as well as build new ones.[32]

Frist Jr. recalled that after the Sunday meeting, he still wasn't convinced that they were "going to do it." Massey and Frist Sr. were worried that their existing obligations would hinder the commitment required to start a new company.[33]

Then, in April 1968, the four men gathered again at the Augusta National Golf Course during the Masters Tournament to "decide whether we're going to do this or not," said Frist Jr. A written study of HCA's first five years succinctly captures what happened next:

What really ensued at Augusta, a natural meeting point for Nashville's leaders who traditionally discuss matters on the greens, was a converging of personalities and motivations. [They] met for two days to compare, to analyze, to examine, to elicit, and to contribute to the far-reaching decision made by Dr. Frist Sr., who said quietly yet succinctly, "Let's do it."[34]

Hospital Corporation of America Is Born

The fledgling company incorporated on May 1, 1968, as Park View Hospital Inc. but changed its name to Hospital Corporation of America in August 1968. At incorporation, it anticipated building, operating, acquiring, and owning acute care facilities.[35] Each man held equal shares. Massey served as chairman of the board and Hooker as vice chairman. Dr. Frist Sr. held the post of president, and Dr. Frist Jr. was executive vice president for medical affairs.

Hospital Corporation of America set up business in May 1968 in this small house in Nashville. The house was located in the parking lot of Park View Hospital. As the company grew, it expanded into trailers.

The company's plan to build and acquire a chain of hospitals was well along when it announced, on June 25, 1968, the acquisition of Park View in a $5 million transaction. The 65 physician-owners swapped their Park View stock for stock in the new corporation. "It took a lot of doing [to convince the doctors]," said Massey. "They had to have confidence in us, or they wouldn't have done the deal."[36]

On the day of Park View's purchase, Massey told the press that Park View was to be the first in a series. Dr. Frist Jr. laid out the company's philosophy and spoke of its ambitious plans. He told the press, "We believe that a corporation, using its experience and combined abilities, can produce significant savings in the architecture, construction, and management of hospitals." He went on to emphasize that each HCA hospital, while maintaining high standards of medical care, would apply management and cost reduction techniques that had been developed and implemented in other industries. Such efficiency would "help combat the spiraling costs of hospitalization," he predicted.[37]

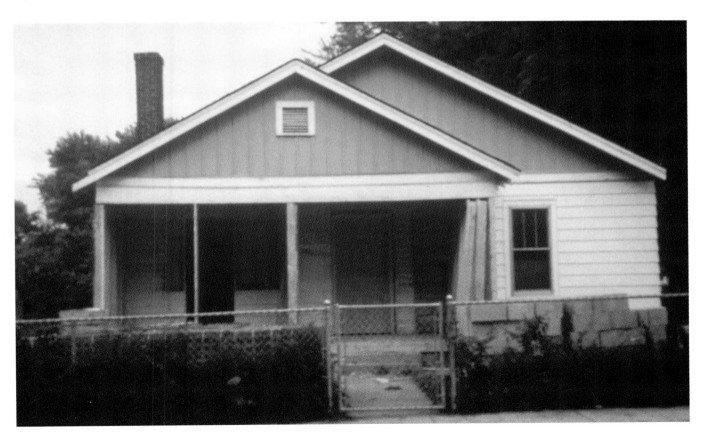

In this letter dated May 2, 1968, Thomas Frist Jr. writes to Sam Fleming, chairman and CEO of Nashville's Third National Bank and owner of the house where the founders met in Augusta: "It now looks as if we are definitely going to incorporate and begin what we hope will be a fine large chain of hospitals around the USA. It is very exciting to think of the fantastic potential; yet on the other hand, a frightening thing to think of the enormity of the undertaking."

Extending Life

In the summer and fall, HCA acquired two existing hospitals in Davidson County (Nashville) and three more elsewhere in the state. It slated new hospitals in Donelson, Erin, Smithville, and Chattanooga, all in Tennessee, and another in Roanoke, Virginia. "We felt the real future was to build hospitals that would be modern and new rather than just to acquire them," said Frist Jr. "That was what led us to Erin, Tennessee, and to Donelson Hospital, where the [doctor owners] had asked my father to help them as a consultant."[38]

For the doctors who had started the hospitals, HCA was a lifeline. Like so many other physician-owners throughout the country, they had reached the point where they needed more capital to keep up with the rising cost of providing quality hospital healthcare.

In Erin, Tennessee, for example, two doctors served a population of 12,000, but there was no hospital where they could admit people in dire need. The physicians and the community had tried valiantly to raise money to build the needed facility but had failed. One of the two doctors then announced that he was leaving; the other said he would go, too, feeling unable to serve so many people by himself. HCA stepped in and built a 36-bed hospital with facilities and services scaled to the size of the community. The two doctors stayed, another arrived, and a board-certified surgeon joined them. The facility in Erin was the first hospital that HCA built and followed a prototype design that Dr. Frist Sr. had used in building the Taylor Hospital in Lewisburg, Tennessee.

Similarly, the owners of the Lewis-Gale Hospital in Roanoke had been thinking about forming a publicly held company consisting of five Virginia hospitals so they could sell shares and secure funds to replace some of the older facilities. David G. Williamson Jr., administrator of Lewis-Gale and one of the owners, contacted Jack Massey because he had heard Massey was leading a similar effort in Nashville. After Frist Jr. evaluated the hospital, HCA made an offer to buy with the understanding that it would build a replacement hospital of at least 200 beds. HCA ended up building a 320-bed hospital with room for an 80-bed expansion.[39]

The physician-owners of Lewis-Gale couldn't have been happier. They received 90,000 shares of HCA stock and got a new hospital in the bargain. As Williamson pointed out, "The main thing the doctors at Lewis-Gale were interested in was securing new facilities. We chose HCA because we were extremely impressed with the quality of the people. They were not in the business to make a fast buck and leave but were committed to quality healthcare, and that was where we were committed."[40]

After the negotiations were complete, Williamson joined HCA's board and went on to become a senior officer at the company and one of its foremost leaders. Williamson was dedicated to providing quality healthcare and was known for his integrity, honesty, and contagious optimism. Frist Jr. once observed that "Dave Williamson embodies the spirit and dedication of the HCA hospital administrator. Through his hospital experience, he has enabled us to maintain our perspective of what is good and necessary for the patient, physician, and community."[41] In fact, Williamson's instinctive leadership skills and ability as an administrator

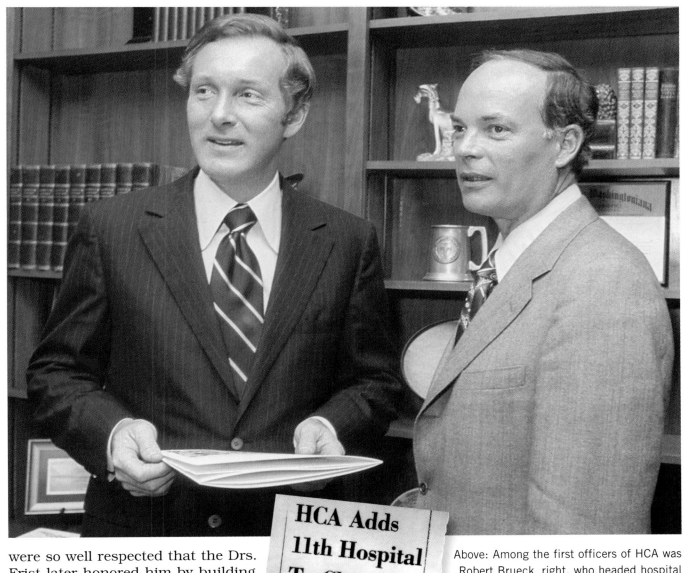

HCA Adds 11th Hospital To Chain

Nashville-based Hospital Corporation of America, which is headed by Jack C. Massey and Dr. Thomas Frist Sr., has purchased the 300-bed Johnson-Willis Hospital in Richmond, Va.

were so well respected that the Drs. Frist later honored him by building the Williamson Room, where hospital administrators could go to work or relax when they visited Nashville headquarters.

Right away, Williamson's contacts in the field of hospital administration introduced HCA to two other Virginia cities: Blacksburg and Pulaski.[42]

By the time construction began on the Donelson facility in late October 1968, the company owned nine others, and plans were in place for building five more in five different states. All acquisitions were accomplished through an exchange of stock with the physicians who owned the facilities.[43]

Above: Among the first officers of HCA was Robert Brueck, right, who headed hospital operations and administrative functions in the early years. He is shown with Thomas Frist Jr., who was executive vice president and responsible for acquisitions and development until 1976, when he took on the additional role of chief operating officer.

Center: HCA owned 10 hospitals toward the end of 1968. This newspaper clipping announces the company's purchase of its 11th— the Johnston-Willis Hospital, a 300-bed facility in Richmond, Virginia. Over the course of the following year, HCA acquired 15 others, bringing the total to 26 at the end of 1969.

Building a Base

For HCA, that first year was one of heavy investment, of building a solid base. Early acquisition and construction took place primarily in rural areas, where healthcare needs were often unmet. As time passed, the company began to see opportunities in suburban locations in mid-size or larger southern cities where the populations were beginning to move away from downtowns. HCA also gravitated to Georgia, Florida, and Texas, where hospitals were strapped for capital to serve all the people moving into the South and Southwest. Many of the doctors who owned these hospitals had been thinking about setting up their own publicly held hospital companies or else joining with one of the other existing hospital chains: American Medical International and National Medical Enterprises, both in California; American Medicorp in Pennsylvania; Extendicare (later Humana) in Kentucky; or Hospital Affiliates International in Nashville. Frist Jr. credited both Massey and Frist Sr. with "creating an aura of excitement" and helping convince the hospitals to join with HCA.[44]

By then Robert P. Brueck had come on board as vice president of administrative affairs. Brueck had proven himself to be a skillful administrator and, in the words of Dr. Frist Sr., was "a gentleman of great integrity."[45] He had worked with Massey at Baptist Hospital and had served as executive director of the Nashville Metropolitan Region Health and Hospital Planning Council.

While Dr. Frist Jr. spent most of his time finding suitable hospitals to acquire or locations to build, Brueck was charged with developing an operational infrastructure. "We moved pretty fast," Brueck remembered of HCA's first years. Between August 1968 and June 1969, HCA acquired 17 hospitals. "But we looked at twice that many," Brueck said. "We weren't satisfied with the medical staff or the facility itself or both.... We didn't want to compromise by taking on hospitals, even if they were available, if they didn't meet our standard of a quality kind of operation."[46]

Though Hospital Corporation of America showed astonishing growth during its first year, that growth didn't come easily. The concept of a private, for-profit company managing a national group of hospitals was a new idea, Jack Massey recalled later. "It was kind of hard to sell the country on it. The biggest problem was getting the money to grow." Going public with stock offerings promised to raise capital needed for HCA's goal of having 100 hospitals in 10 years, but the founders had to guess what a share should sell for.

"For about a year we had been buying hospitals using lettered stock for which we had put an arbitrary value on of $25," Massey said. "We'd buy a hospital by trading stock that we thought was worth $25."

"I think a key factor that made all this possible ...was being able to trade stock in a company that really wasn't publicly held," said Frist Jr. "One of the reasons we were able to do this was that Park View shareholders during this "go-go" glamorous period in the market sold the stock they had received in HCA in private transactions to people outside of their group.... Each time we would make an acquisition, a new benchmark would be created, and they would sell their stock at a higher level. So by having the stock to trade with, we did not have a need for cash."[47]

Indeed, revenues at the end of 1968 reached $29 million, and after-tax earnings crossed the $1 million mark. That's when the founders knew it was time for an IPO (initial public offering).[48]

Public Prestige

On March 4, 1969, the New York investment banking firm Goodbody & Company took HCA public. With so many speculative schemes taking advantage of the hot stock market, the firm was all too happy to underwrite HCA. James G. Leonard, Goodbody's head of investment, remembered thinking of HCA as "the Tiffany of the medical care organizations."[49]

Massey had learned at Kentucky Fried Chicken that it was a good strategy to set a public offering price that would be fair to the company yet low enough to ensure that shareholders were happy from the start. (Massey would later tell HCA Senior Vice President Vic Campbell that shareholders are business partners and companies should do everything within reason to keep them happy.) Buyers thought that HCA would open at $25, but instead Massey priced it at $18. By the end of the day, the

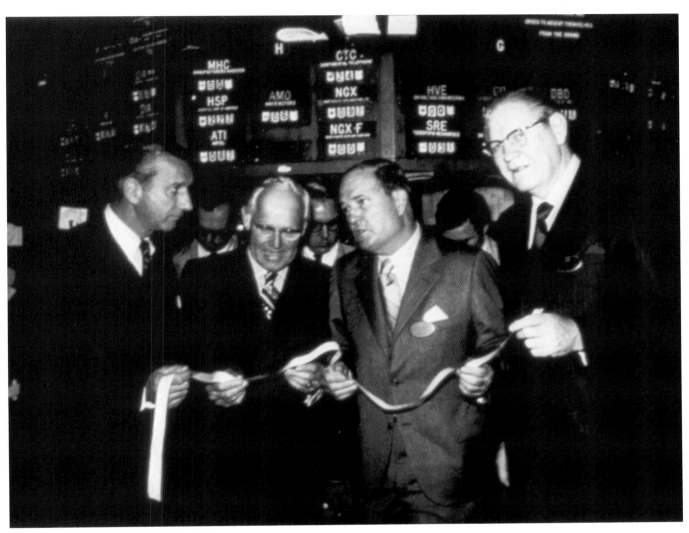

In November 1970, Hospital Corporation of America was listed on the New York Stock Exchange, broadening the market for its securities. Shown here (starting second from left) are Chairman Jack Massey, President John Hill, and Vice Chairman Thomas Frist Sr.

stock had soared to $46, with 400,000 shares sold, and the IPO had raised $7.2 million.[50]

Now, with a publicly traded stock, it was easier to agree on valuations with sellers of hospitals. By the end of its first year as a public company, with 26 hospitals housing more than 3,000 beds, HCA had become the nation's largest group of investor-owned hospitals.

Some of the early acquisitions came about because the doctor-owners personally knew the senior Dr. Frist and held him in high regard. As Frist Jr. said of his father in 1976, "Even without his knowing it, people came to us whom he had trained at Vanderbilt or Saint Thomas—people he had known through medical meetings, medical benevolence foundations, and medical missionary work. It was surprising how many of these relationships dating back 15, 20, and 30 years would benefit HCA in its formative years."[51]

Others studied what Kentucky Fried Chicken had done, and they expected Jack Massey to take HCA to similar heights. Few were disappointed in that regard; those who had sold their hospitals to the company at $25 a share soon found themselves wealthy. And 20 years after the company's founding, an original share of HCA stock was worth about $186.[52]

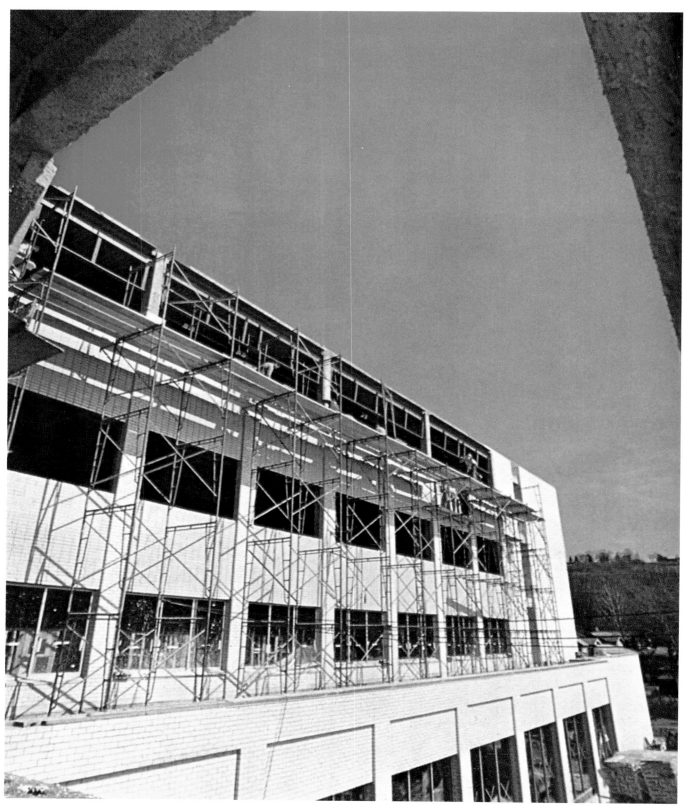

The company's first 200-bed hospital rises in Chattanooga, Tennessee. Two other identical hospitals were built that same year, in Macon and Albany, Georgia.

CHAPTER TWO

BUILDING A BALANCE SHEET AND A MANAGEMENT TEAM

1970 – 1973

There is a growing awareness of the importance of the private sector in the nation's healthcare delivery system and increasing receptivity toward our concepts and our methods.

—Jack Massey and John Hill, 1971

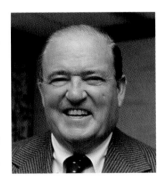

ONCE HCA BECAME A PUBLICLY traded company, it had a much easier time acquiring hospitals using stock as payment. But to ensure that it could meet the growing opportunities to build new hospitals, the company held a secondary offering of 500,000 shares in September 1970. In November 1970, HCA stock was listed on the New York Stock Exchange (NYSE). Many so-called hot stocks of the 1960s had not lived up to investors' expectations, and the NYSE listing helped establish HCA's credibility as a company that would be around for the long term.[1]

The company grew beyond anyone's wildest dreams, due in no small part to the gifted judgments of both Drs. Frist and Jack Massey. (Henry Hooker resigned from HCA in 1969, before HCA's IPO, to focus his energy on various family business ventures.) To better manage the sprawling enterprise they had begun, the three entrepreneurs recruited a remarkable set of energetic, ambitious executives, some young, some seasoned.

Building a Team

Clearly, the young company needed to broaden its management team. Up until 1970, Dr. Frist Sr. had been HCA's president, but his active medical practice and the company's rapid growth led the three founders to seek someone who had

experience in running a major company and who could focus full-time on HCA and the new hospital industry. That March, the board elected John A. Hill, 62, as president of HCA.

Frist Sr. recalled that Hill had some misgivings about taking the job because he thought Frist Sr. might resent his coming as a replacement. "I reassured him very quickly that it would be the greatest blessing for me to have a man of his stature and experience and wisdom to replace me," said Frist Sr. "It was a great day in my life when he came. My ego doesn't depend on titles."[2]

Born in Oklahoma, Hill graduated from the University of Denver in 1928 and joined the Denver office of Aetna Life Insurance Company. He spent a career working his way up through the ranks, becoming president in 1962. He had just taken early retirement from Aetna when he joined HCA's board in February 1970. As a respected businessman, he brought national credibility to HCA. Hill opened many doors with lenders and analysts and helped establish basic management operational procedures.[3]

John Hill was elected president of HCA effective April 1, 1970. He succeeded Thomas Frist Sr., who became the company's vice chairman of the board and chief medical officer.

"I've been blessed with many mentors over the years, and John Hill was one of the most important ones," said Dr. Frist Jr. more than 30 years later. "Dad gave me common sense, quality, the humanistic approach to running a business, but John Hill gave me my college degree. He brought something of great value to a group of young management folks who were not nearly as experienced as he was. From his years at Aetna, he brought great sales and marketing experience as well as a tremendous network of relationships with corporate America. He was a cultured individual who was an avid collector of western art. He and his wife, Margaret, served as wonderful role models for a young management team."[4]

The company drew another important early executive from the insurance field. At the age of 54, John C. Neff joined HCA in 1968 as chief financial officer. Neff was largely responsible for raising capital and developing relationships with HCA's long-term lenders. Born in Chicago, he earned a master's degree in business administration following service in World War II. After a stint at Merrill Lynch, Pierce, Fenner, and Smith, he joined State Farm Mutual, then became financial vice president at Nashville-based Life and Casualty Insurance Company. He had recently cofounded an investment services company with Massey when the HCA founders recruited him.[5]

Another financial guru, Sam A. Brooks Jr., joined HCA in 1969 as senior controller. Brooks had been an auditor at Ernst and Ernst in Dallas and quickly became Neff's right-hand man. He and Neff helped the company through some difficult financial challenges after the U.S. stock market plummeted in May 1970.[6]

Donald W. Fish joined HCA in March 1970 to start an in-house legal department. Within a year he had been promoted to vice president, secretary, and general counsel. Fish described his early years at the company as one of constantly shifting priorities. "Priorities frequently changed, several times in the course of a week or maybe even in the course of a day," he said. "And I don't think that my experience in that regard was anything unusual. I think we all had frequent changes of priorities, but the need to obtain and to finalize the company's long-term financing and the need to compete effectively in the acquisition area were probably two of our most pressing interests."[7]

These management appointments were strategic ones. Borrowing money was key to building hospitals and a difficult challenge in the case of for-profit hospitals since the hospital industry was virtually a not-for-profit business. The experience of Hill, Neff, Brooks, and Fish and Jack Massey's business stature opened doors in the financial community that were essential not only to HCA's future but to the entire investor-owned hospital industry.

"Securing financing was one of the most important and challenging aspects of getting the company started," said Fish, who assisted in the company's negotiations for financing. "In all candor, we were not in much of a position in those days to dictate terms; we accepted the major terms that were offered to us. But we were able to negotiate some of the more significant restrictive terms they proposed."[8]

Instead of financing projects one by one, HCA borrowed large sums from banks and institutional investors to fund a group of hospitals. "The lending institutions weren't too eager to make a loan on a large hospital because hospitals in general had not

Left: Sam Brooks, who served 16 years with the company, joined HCA in 1969 as senior controller and later became HCA's CFO. He retired in 1994.

Right: Don Fish started with HCA in 1970 and a year later was promoted to vice president, general counsel, and secretary.

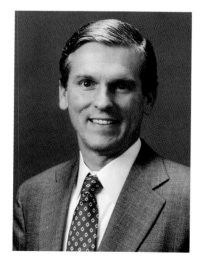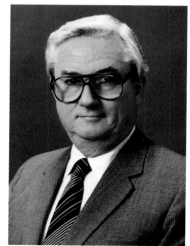

been managed very well," said Brooks, who in 1973 became the company's CFO. "The lenders had to be sold on the economic viability of hospitals. Also, we had the added benefit of not making a loan on one large hospital but making a loan on several hospitals. They were able to spread their risk."[9]

"Mortgage loan packages like we did had never been done before," said John Neff. But just as important as the package financing, he added, was encouraging lenders to agree to let HCA finance additions on the hospital without having to pay off the original loan. "This was terribly important," he said. "Hospitals are constantly expanding, and if we had to refinance the hospital every time we expanded—take it out of the package and go finance it somewhere else—it would have been impossible."[10]

None of HCA's competitors had been able to pool hospitals into a loan package, and many saw their growth falter as a result. "The competition had such trouble because we were swamping the market," said Neff. "We worked hard at getting acquainted with these lenders. We prided ourselves on the fact that we always did what we said we would do, so when we went for more money, we were never a problem loan to anybody."[11]

Neff pointed out that some lending institutions were happy to lend money to HCA because they saw the venture as something of a crusade. "They were doing something that had never been done before," said Neff, "lending to companies that were showing the hospital industry that private enterprise could do a good job."[12]

Nashville's First American, Third National, and Commerce Union offered a loan on the condition that First National City Bank of New York join the venture. Massey, Hill, and Neff went to see officials there. For a while it looked as if National City Bank were going to back away. Then Massey took the floor, saying, "You don't have any relationship with anyone in the hospital field or in the medical field. Don't you want to be the first one in it? Don't you want to lead out and get the business of this company as it grows?" In July 1970 First National City Bank did indeed "lead out," sealing the consortium's deal for $30 million. A group of eight insurance companies loaned the company $27 million in 1972, and another bank consortium put up $35 million in 1974.[13]

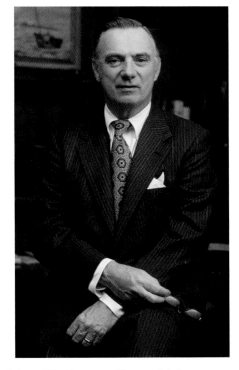

John Neff originally served as treasurer of HCA, then vice president of finance and executive vice president. In 1972 he became president, a post he held until 1976.

"The insurance companies have been good to us," Massey once observed. "They give us what we want because we provide 40 percent of our construction costs out of cash flow." HCA's competitors, he observed, "haven't realized the necessity of maintaining the proper relationship with the credit world." Even so, HCA remained a highly leveraged company, with about 60 percent of its capitalization in long-term debt—but leveraging was not undesirable, because cash flow in the hospital business was very predictable.[14]

Other funds came through secondary stock offerings during the 1970s. The company also reinvested its earnings in more facilities. Finally, a small number of projects were financed through local revenue bond issues.

John Hill acknowledged that money was tight in those early years, and it didn't help that HCA was considered "a young company without a great deal of standing."[15] It is a testament to the skill, experience, and perseverance of the founders, Hill, and HCA's other leaders that the company was able to grow as quickly as it did.

Excellent Operations

After quality patient care, the chief goal of HCA management was the sound operation of company hospitals. "After we acquired about 11 hospitals, we became more concerned with coordinating the administrative affairs of those hospitals," said Bob Brueck. "We had decided early in the game

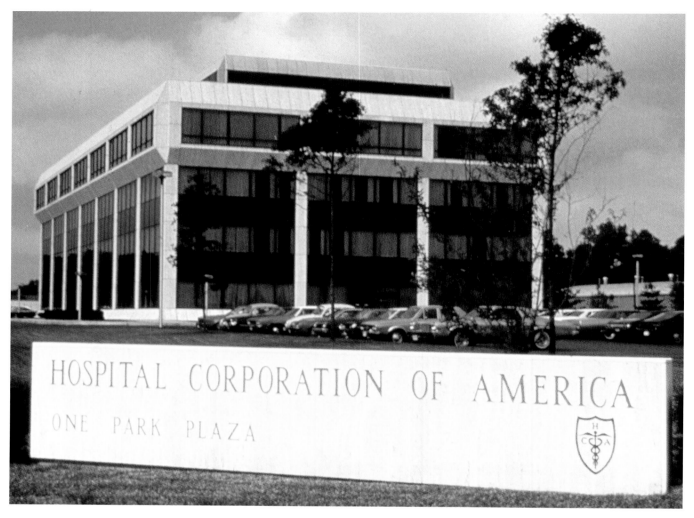

In December 1972, HCA moved into its new corporate headquarters building near its original hospital, Park View, in Nashville. Initially about half of the space in the four-story building was leased to other tenants.

that we would operate with a highly decentralized philosophy. Running a hospital is highly personalized. When people go into the hospitals, they are not interested in being treated like everyone else. [Similarly], I think it's important that the local physicians and administrators and nurses look on their activities as being very personalized."[16]

Each hospital's local physicians and staff were fully responsible for medical, professional, and ethical oversight activities. The frontline management team comprised a professional hospital administrator, an experienced financial officer, and a director of nursing. They worked in cooperation with a local board of trustees made up of civic leaders and physicians drawn from the community.[17]

Wherever it could, the company introduced automated, labor-saving devices such as patient-monitoring equipment. Electrocardiograms were

transmitted by telephone from small hospitals to large ones and read by experts, who returned a report in minutes. Centralization of accounting jobs, especially the complicated Medicare and Medicaid accounts, eliminated the need for each hospital to have its own accounting department.

Nashville headquarters provided central personnel services, giving all company hospitals the services of dieticians, technicians in pathology and radiology, inhalation therapists, and medical librarians. Support services that would otherwise have to be bought locally at great expense came from headquarters at significant savings and included services of attorneys, auditors, public relations counselors, employee communications staff, data processors, and others. This centralization held down costs while providing technical help that would have been beyond the means of the smaller institutions in the HCA family.

From the beginning, HCA achieved major savings through large-scale centralized purchasing of equipment and supplies. Where an individual hospital got discounts of 30 to 35 percent on supplies, vice president Robert C. Crosby, who joined HCA in 1969, estimated that HCA got group discounts of 60 to 65 percent.[18]

Buying insurance coverage for HCA hospitals as a group slashed hefty premiums. HCA's architects designed standard buildings in four basic sizes that could be constructed at any future location and expanded to keep pace with community needs. HCA built its new facilities according to a critical-path method, buying materials for several construction projects at once at favorable prices.

Economy of operation factored into site selection, too. HCA tended to build in clusters. A large "mother hospital" might be at the hub of several smaller ones within 40 to 50 miles. The large facility did the routine laboratory tests and dietary work for the small units, and it was also home base for the helicopter that shuttled the pathologists and dieticians among the sites.[19]

All hospitals were of masonry, steel, and glass construction, designed for long life and minimum maintenance. The standardized design and equipment led to shorter construction periods, lower borrowing and building costs, and a reduction in the time it took to achieve profitable operations. This was a particular advantage for the rapidly growing HCA in the 1970s, when inflation and cost of capital were in double digits.[20]

This overall sameness on the outside did not lead to drabness on the inside. Patient rooms were carpeted and had private baths, color television, individual control for temperature and humidity, and electric beds. Patients entering the door of HCA's West Paces Ferry Hospital, in Atlanta, might have felt they were checking into an expensive hotel that, in addition to the above amenities, offered a dozen entrees for dinner. Such amenities would one day become commonplace in hospitals but weren't necessarily widespread in the early 1970s.[21]

Quality without Compromise

Some of HCA's critics assumed that lower costs would compromise the quality of care. But the management of HCA knew that high-quality care could harmonize with lower costs. The company sought to provide every acute and support service any patient needed—but at the same time to make

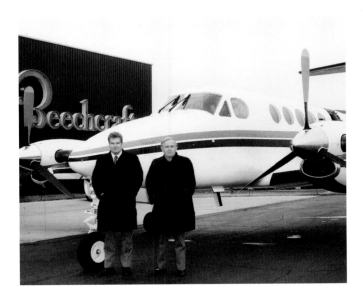

HCA's first corporate pilots pose with a 1975 Beechcraft Super King Air 200. Glenn Mitchell (right) was a retired air force lieutenant colonel who served as an instructor pilot in the 65th Bomb Wing with Dr. Frist Jr. He piloted for HCA from 1969 to 2000. Gaylord Dorn (left) started piloting for HCA in 1971 and was senior pilot in 2003. Aviation played a key role in HCA's development and growth. In the late 1960s and early 1970s, Dr. Frist Jr., an ATP-rated pilot, flew a Piper Aztec from Nashville to small towns and cities (most of which did not have commercial airports) throughout the Southeast and Southwest to meet with doctors and community leaders about the prospect of HCA buying their local hospitals or building new ones to meet growing healthcare needs. In the mid-1990s, Jack Bovender joined Dr. Frist Jr. as a multiengine-instrument-and-commercial-rated pilot.

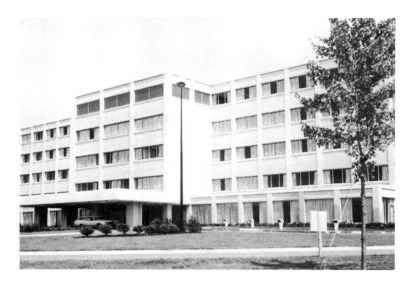

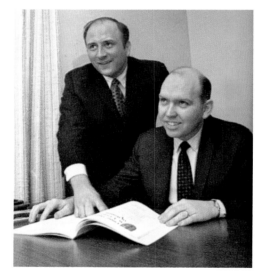

every dollar in plant, physician, and operating costs do its utmost. HCA was bringing proven business principles from other economic sectors to the hospital business, which, for the most part, had been run like a cottage industry.[22]

HCA liked to cite the Johnston-Willis Hospital in Richmond, Virginia, as exemplifying its best methods. Acquired in 1968, the not-for-profit Johnston-Willis was one of the company's first purchases, and the 50-year-old institution looked rather dowdy. It was making $3.07 per patient per day when HCA purchased it. By 1976 HCA had raised that figure to $6.36, mainly through bulk purchasing and shared employees and equipment. Services were not cut; indeed, J-W (as local people called it) gained a reputation for the best emergency room in the city, with fast admission and lab services and the newest equipment.

J-W was also a good place to evaluate the criticism of for-profit hospitals: that they shifted the burdens of treating the poor and training

Upper left: Chippenham Hospital, a 204-bed facility serving a suburban section of Richmond, Virginia, opened in 1972.

Left: Paul McKnight (standing), who joined HCA as personnel director in 1969, served the company for 26 years, the last several as head of group operations in Florida.

Below: In 1971 HCA acquired the 223-bed Los Robles Hospital in Thousand Oaks, California, a Los Angeles suburb.

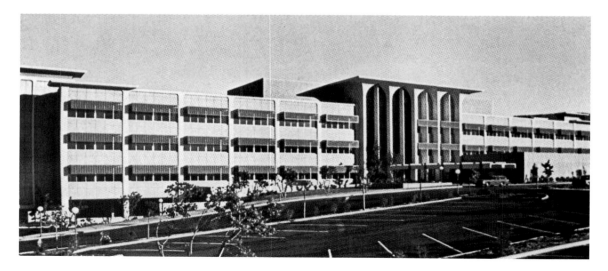

physicians to nonprofit and government hospitals. On the contrary, anyone who arrived at J-W— or any other HCA hospital over the company's 35 years—would not be turned away. HCA has always offered charitable services at its hospitals, with the figures for uncompensated care totaling about $2 billion per year by 2003. As for doctor training, J-W administrator John Tobin Jr. pointed out in 1976 that the hospital paid real estate and corporate income taxes that helped support Richmond's public Medical College of Virginia Hospital.[23]

Symbolic of HCA's dedication to quality patient care was the Dr. Thomas F. Frist Sr. Humanitarian Award. The bronze statue, which depicts Dr. Frist with his arms sheltering two children, was first awarded in 1972 to Janis Buchanan, a nursing assistant at Palm Drive Hospital in Sebastapol, California. Buchanan was judged "most compassionate," and by awarding her the statue, HCA demonstrated its readiness to reward individual initiative as well as its commitment to the welfare of the patient.

South ... West

HCA's earliest acquisitions and construction projects were in the South. One reason for this, Brueck noted, was proximity to HCA's Nashville headquarters. "Besides that, the more industrialized sections of the country, and the Northeast, for example, had the Metcalf-McCluskey law, which prohibited our kind of operation. They also had higher prices, union problems, and other kinds of difficulties in obtaining people."[24]

Many towns and cities had voluntary, proprietary, or publicly owned general hospitals serving mainly surgical and obstetrical patients and deliberately foregoing specialized technology. Although small, the hospitals provided employment for local people and volunteer opportunities for others. They also allowed patients to be treated near their homes. When Dr. Frist Sr. spoke of the absence of "happy attitudes" in hospitals, he may have accurately described large urban research and teaching institutions, but for small-town America, the hospital was a relatively cheerful institution with legions of volunteers. Young women joined the Candy Stripers, and "Gray Ladies," a service unit the Red Cross started in World War I, helped make

sure that veterans were as comfortable as possible during their time in the hospital.[25]

As the South experienced an influx of people during the late 1960s and early 1970s, the need for more and better hospitals became apparent. In its first years, HCA was invited to build new hospitals in many more communities than it was able to. In some cases, the company was able to help a locality build or upgrade a hospital when the area otherwise would have done without.

The twin communities of Blacksburg and Christiansburg, Virginia, for example, had one small, antiquated hospital between them. The facility still used a hand-cranked elevator to transport patients. The towns' leaders applied for Hill-Burton funds on three separate occasions and were turned down. They attempted a public subscription drive, but it fell far short. The communities were saved when HCA opened a modern facility to serve them.[26]

The year 1971 was memorable as HCA slipped its southern identity and went west, purchasing Ross Medical Corporation, a California company

In 1971 HCA entered the hospital market in California with a bang. The company acquired Ross Medical Corporation, with its chain of four hospitals in the San Francisco area, including the 44-bed Palm Drive Hospital in Sebastapol, shown here.

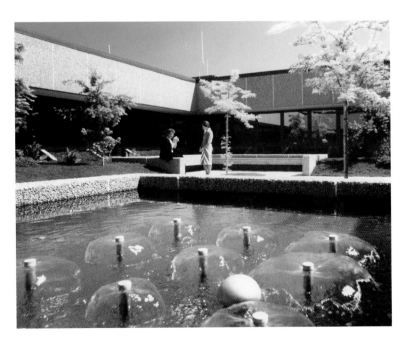

PHYSICIAN RELATIONS

THE PRINCIPAL CONCERN OF PHYSI-
cians is to provide quality patient care,
and HCA has done everything possible to
ensure that its hospitals do just that. Many of
HCA's hospitals were acquired from groups of
doctors who had started them to fill a local need
for a facility where they could treat their patients.
As healthcare became more expensive, mainly as
a result of advancing technology, the doctors
found they could no longer afford to provide the
best possible service—but they saw that HCA
could. Though HCA hospitals' physicians did not
share in ownership of its hospitals, they did participate in determining the hospitals' policies,
services, and equipment.[1]

From its founding, HCA recognized the
importance of establishing good relationships
with physicians, and the staff of its various hospitals worked hard to give doctors the best possible service and assistance. Doctors' offices, for
example, were constructed near or in every HCA
hospital. Moreover, each hospital was largely
directed by doctors on a local board of trustees
that was responsible for the hospital's policies.[2]
In the 1960s and 1970s, most hospitals in the
country did not allow physicians to serve on their
board of trustees. Frist Sr., however, insisted that
the board of trustees of every HCA hospital have
significant physician representation.[3] (Today,
most U.S. hospitals follow this practice.)

In 1972 John Hill organized a board of
governors, comprising physicians from communities HCA served, to advise the company on
patient care issues. The panel, under the chair-
manship of Dr. Frist Sr., advised management
on methods of recruiting personnel and particularly on filling shortages in specific areas. It
also monitored social and governmental developments that might impact patient care.
Finally, the governors made recommendations
on medical and technical innovations for
company hospitals.[4]

Perhaps George Mercy best
summed up HCA's philosophy
regarding doctors when he said,
"A hospital is an empty, useless
building without physician support.
The physicians are the ones who
admit the patients, so you need
the physician support and the
physician confidence in the company and in the facility." He added
that Dr. Frist Sr. and Dr. Frist Jr.
played a huge role in inspiring just
such confidence.[5]

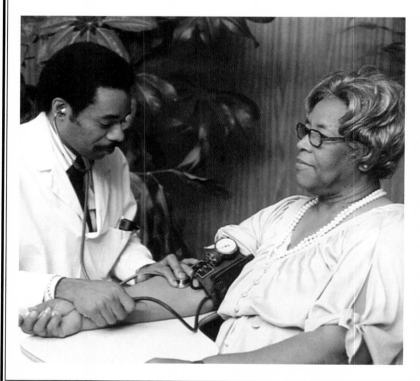

Dr. Frank Royal, a practicing physician
in Richmond, Virginia, served on HCA's
Board of Governors, which advised
management on medical and professional
matters, in 1979. Royal would later
join HCA's board of directors and still
served on the board in 2003.

with four hospitals that gave HCA a foothold in San Francisco, another growing region. A year later the company bought four more hospitals in or near San Francisco, one in Los Angeles, and another in a growing suburb of Portland, Oregon.

After HCA acquired Ross Medical, Vice President C. George Mercy was placed in charge of the new Western Division of HCA operations. Mercy had come to HCA's board in 1969 after the company acquired Houston's Diagnostic Center Hospital, where he had been administrator, executive director, and chairman of the board. He began working full time at HCA in 1971 and within a year had demonstrated his abilities not only in management but also in finance, acquisitions, and accounting.[27] Mercy is considered one of the pioneers of HCA; his wise counsel and dedication to improving healthcare were instrumental in the company's success.

By the end of 1971, the company operated 40 hospitals housing 5,250 beds in 12 states, a gain of 12 facilities and 2,100 beds in a single year. Unquestionably, management's pride was justified when the press and investors declared that Hospital Corporation of America had become the dominant force in the nation's proprietary hospital business.[28]

Gaining Credibility

In its early days, HCA struggled to bring credibility to the for-profit hospital industry. If some writers, regulators, and politicians looked askance at "hospitals for profit," others took the company to task for "cream skimming"—that is, providing only services with high profit margins and omitting amenities like emergency rooms and obstetrics. The accusations were unfounded. HCA designed its suburban hospitals to cater to the needs of young couples having children, for example, and by the early 1970s, emergency rooms were universally required for licensure.[29]

Others unfriendly to the company raised questions about HCA's relationship with physicians. Management replied that local doctors who served on an HCA hospital board were not obliged to refer their patients to that hospital, and they cited examples of many doctors who did not. And

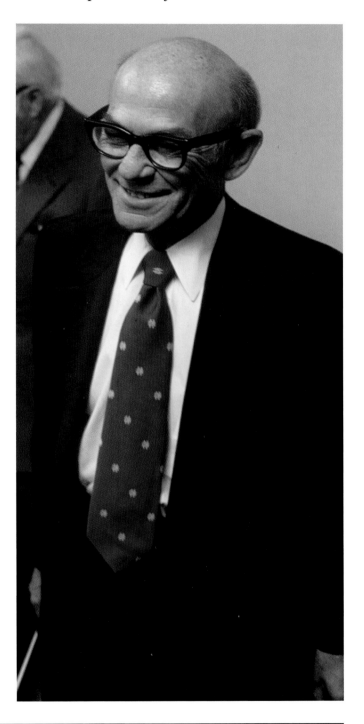

C. George Mercy, former executive director of Diagnostic Center Hospital in Houston, Texas, was named vice president in charge of West Coast operations and was elected to the executive committee in 1971.

while individual physicians could buy stock in the company, just as they could in any publicly traded business, they could not buy ownership in a hospital. No staff physician at an HCA hospital had any direct ownership or share in its profits.[30]

Company operations took on a new dimension in 1972 when communities began asking HCA to replace existing nonprofit hospitals with investor-owned facilities. "At first it was very difficult to convince people that we should be allowed to replace a hospital," said Sam Brooks. "But once our business reputation for delivering a quality product had become established, and because we could get the money, we were being invited to replace not-for-profit hospitals."[31]

In Frankfort, Kentucky, a newly constructed HCA hospital replaced a tax-exempt one. In two Tennessee communities, the company's new facility replaced city-county hospitals, and in Pulaski, Virginia, an HCA hospital took the place of a voluntary community hospital.[32]

By proposing to build new hospitals that actually paid taxes rather than draining them, HCA quickly caught the attention of beleaguered planning boards and city managers.

Milton Johnson, who began working for HCA in 1980 and by 1999 had become HCA's controller and senior vice president, pointed out that investor-owned hospital companies could do more for the community than not-for-profits. "Not-for-profits have to do more than break even," he said. "They have to generate a reasonable profit to reinvest because of the technology changes that occur in healthcare. When HCA comes into a community, we pay property tax, sales taxes, income taxes. This provides a whole new tax

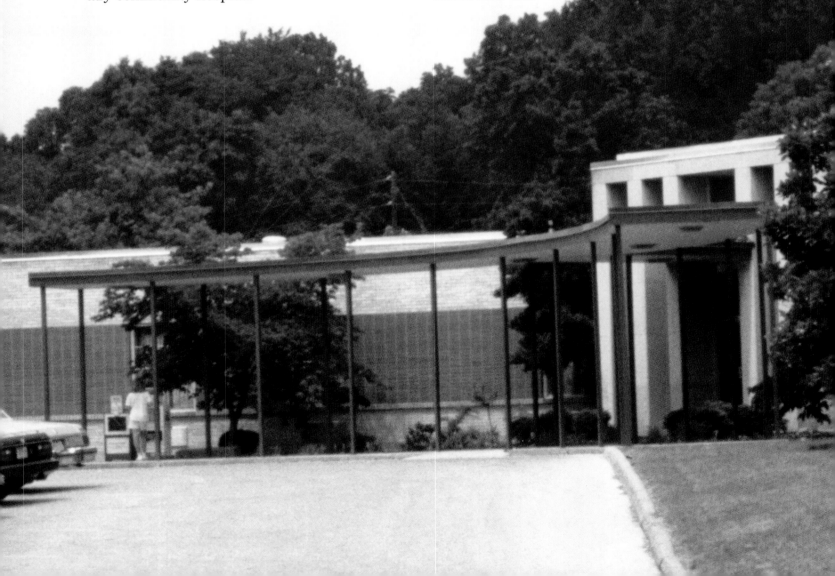

base to fund schools, healthcare, and other programs in those communities."[33]

In towns where HCA built new hospitals, the company became not only a taxpayer but also a major employer, a customer of local businesses, and a participant in local affairs. In some small towns, the HCA hospital was the biggest building and the largest employer. HCA administrators encouraged their employees to take part in civic endeavors, and company hospitals sponsored first-aid and lifesaving courses, offered drug abuse lectures, and held blood drives.[34]

At larger HCA facilities, doctors could take advantage of professional development offerings to satisfy continuing education requirements. The company established other educational programs,

Trinity Hospital in Erin, Tennessee, with 36 beds, was HCA's smallest holding in 1969. One of the first facilities constructed by HCA, Trinity was even smaller than the company's smallest prototypes.

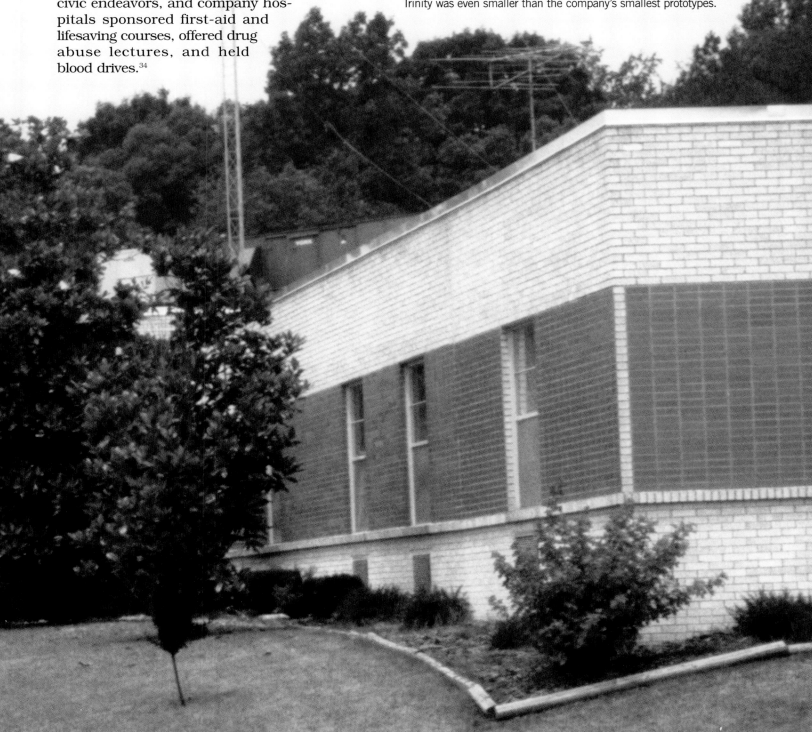

including a full-scale residency program for newly minted physicians at one large hospital, and preceptor relationships with three schools offering degrees in hospital administration.[35]

As HCA became better known, Johnson said, competing with not-for-profits became more and more acceptable "because we were HCA. It was a positive thing because the communities knew we were going to have a fabulous physical plant for healthcare. We attracted quality physicians and provided very good care."[36]

HCA also attracted quality hospital administrators and staff. "We had a great deal of interest on the part of administrators who liked our concept," said Brueck. "Therefore, a number of very good applicants were available."[37] Once HCA found a good administrator, that person selected a controller and director of nursing and department heads, who in turn hired other employees. As Dr. Frist Sr. noted, "The hospital administrator is the key to our success." Frist Sr. took the time to interview each of HCA's potential administrators "because once you get a good administrator, he begets other good people. Good people beget good people."[38]

Government Relations

In early 1971, John Hill was appointed by President Richard Nixon to the Health Care Services Committee of the Cost of Living Council, which

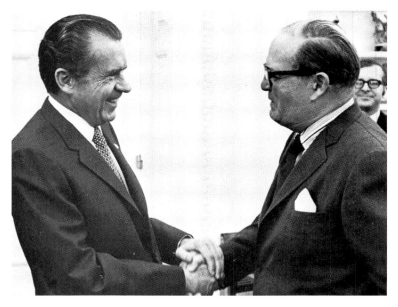

developed guidelines under the administration's wage-and-price-control program. Hill was chosen to represent the for-profit hospital industry; the 12-member committee included representatives of such organizations as the American Hospital Association, the American Medical Association, and the American Pharmaceutical Association. "That might have been one of the most interesting and traumatic series of events that I've ever been through," said Hill. "I was particularly unpopular because no one knew anything about the for-profit hospital industry, and they were very suspicious of it." After a trying three months, however, Hill said that "all of a sudden, HCA and the for-profit industry began to receive a lot of credit and a lot of prestige."[39] Overall, the committee was very successful in holding down healthcare costs—perhaps too successful, according to Hill. After the price controls ended, healthcare prices skyrocketed to try to compensate for the years with restrictions.

HCA foresaw the continuing and looming presence of Washington in medicine. HCA Vice

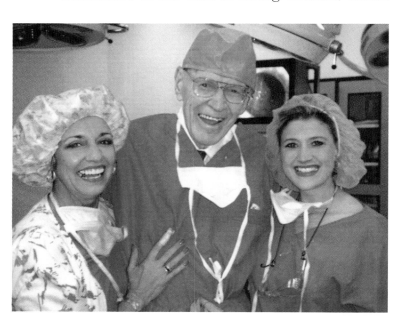

Above: President Richard Nixon discusses activities of the Heath Care Services Committee with John Hill. Nixon appointed Hill to the special committee.

Left: Dr. Frist Sr.'s encouraging and caring presence inspired everyone who knew him.

President James F. Hughes actively contacted members of Congress and their staffs to present HCA's views on the scope and content of various national health insurance proposals. And in 1973 the company opened a government-relations office in Washington, D.C., under the direction of Dave Williamson.

Williamson determined that HCA should not compete with organizations that sought to manage healthcare costs but instead should develop a total corporate response to such third-party organizations as the American Insurance Association and Blue Cross. Later he was appointed president of the Federation of American Hospitals, which

THE GOVERNMENT ENTERS HEALTHCARE IN A BIG WAY

MEDICARE IS A NATIONAL HEALTH insurance program for people over 65 or with serious disabilities. Enacted by Congress in 1965, it was the centerpiece of President Lyndon Johnson's "Great Society" program. Franklin D. Roosevelt had proposed far-reaching health insurance benefits when Social Security was created 30 years before. Organized medicine and private insurance companies had opposed this part of Roosevelt's plan and continued to lead the fight against national health insurance through the 1940s and 1950s.

The Kerr-Mills Act, passed by Congress in 1960, provided federal support for state healthcare programs that served poor elderly people, but eligibility was limited, and the matching-grant formula meant that the poorest states often received the least assistance.

Lawmakers and policy analysts continued to ponder whether

a federal health insurance program should be open to rich and poor alike. They also contemplated the role the states should play. In the end, Medicare was designed as a grand compromise. All persons of age were eligible, regardless of their incomes, and the federal government would administer the program. Meanwhile, Medicaid would serve only poor people, and its management would be given to the states.

Finally, the private sector, from which opposition to national health insurance had come, was guaranteed a major role: Recipients of Medicare would purchase all their services from a provider of their own choosing. The program gave millions of older people and disabled people new access to medical care.[1]

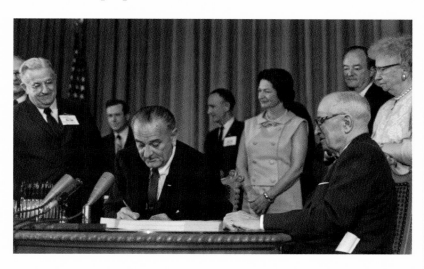

President Lyndon B. Johnson signs the Medicare bill into law while former President Harry Truman (seated, right), also a proponent of national health insurance, watches. Medicare provided American senior citizens with hospital and medical insurance, regardless of their financial means. *(Image courtesy LBJ Library.)*

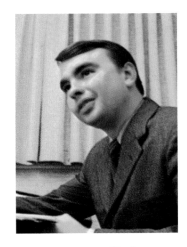

John Colton, one of HCA's first corporate employees in 1968, rose through the ranks over his 27 years with HCA to become a senior vice president of group operations.

was heavily involved in government relations with an emphasis on investor-owned hospitals.[40]

Federal government policy was rapidly becoming the most powerful force in the growth and development of American hospitals. Certificate-of-need regulations, the 1972 Medicare amendments, and what HCA termed the "harsh restrictions" of the price-control program all required that HCA make its voice heard in the nation's capital.[41]

Contract Management

In 1970 HCA began a program of operating hospitals for other owners, beginning with a contract to manage North Shore Hospital in Miami. "They were very eager to have us come in and take over the operation of their hospital, but they did not want to sell their hospital," Brueck remembered. "We were interested in trying it just to see what was involved in the management of hospitals for other owners. So we developed a contract."[42] Bob Crosby was assigned to North Shore, and the company quickly boosted the quality of the Miami hospital's patient care and put it back on its financial feet. The entire affair was a learning experience for HCA, and other management contracts followed.[43]

Management contracts could be negotiated in a matter of weeks while construction of a new hospital took two years or more—and management contracts required no capital outlays. HCA typically could save its client hospitals 10 to 30 percent on purchasing through buying in bulk. HCA offered management systems to keep track of receivables and costs and had platoons of specialists in such areas as Medicare and insurance reimbursement. It also offered computer services to help the hospitals run more efficiently. A management contract usually ran from three to five years, and the fee amounted to 6 or 7 percent of the hospital's revenues. Management contracts became a non-capital-intensive strategy of diversification for HCA.

The company managed hospitals owned by others in much the same way that it ran its own, placing primary responsibility on three key personnel: the administrator, the head of nursing, and the controller. And it turned chronic money losers into financially stable operations. For example, when HCA took over management of Holy Family Hospital in Spokane, Washington, in 1973, the 200-bed institution had lost $650,000 in the previous year. It could pay its nurses only half of a promised 10 percent raise, and accounting was taking up to four months to collect accounts receivable. HCA replaced the hospital's giant IBM 370 computer with its own system, and the average daily computer cost per patient dropped from $12 to $2.25. HCA also cut receivables to an average of 60 days.

With its national purchasing power, HCA saved Holy Family $100,000 in the contract's first year. The nurses received their back pay and got a 12 percent raise. The hospital raised its rates only 8 percent in the process—half the nationwide inflation rate in hospital costs at the time—and paid HCA a fee of $300,000.

In addition to managing existing hospitals, HCA offered to develop new ones for other owners, carrying projects from conception to the "turning of the key" (turnkey contracts). It could carry out feasibility studies, select a site, do the architectural and engineering work, build the hospital, equip it—and manage it under contract.[44]

Saudi Arabia

HCA's leaders began to study international business opportunities as a possible diversification effort while staying within its core business of being a healthcare company. As early as the spring of 1972, HCA President John Hill had told the *Wall Street Journal* that the company was considering starting Latin American and European operations,[45] and George Mercy kept busy as a one-man evaluation team reviewing international opportunities in Greece, France, and Spain.[46]

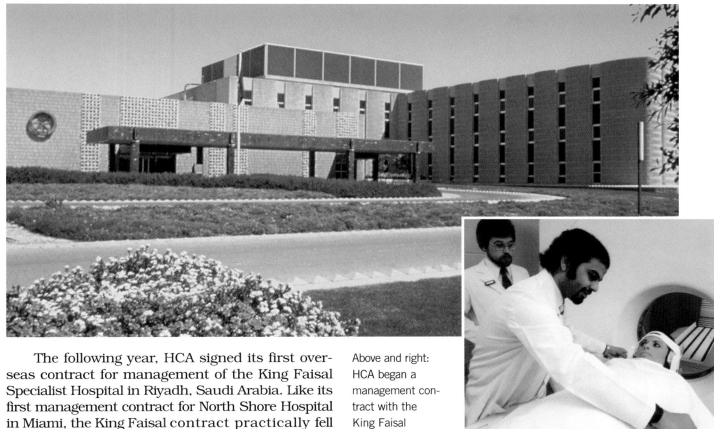

The following year, HCA signed its first overseas contract for management of the King Faisal Specialist Hospital in Riyadh, Saudi Arabia. Like its first management contract for North Shore Hospital in Miami, the King Faisal contract practically fell in HCA's lap. "Somebody contacted us because we were the industry leader, and people call the leader," said Bob Crosby.[47]

King Faisal wanted to build a model hospital and healthcare center—a facility that all the country's other healthcare centers would strive to emulate. To accomplish this, the king hired his personal physician, Dr. Rifat Alsayed Ali, and to give the project more flexibility, excused it from adhering to royal decrees and laws. It was Dr. Rifat who felt the hospital needed the best management in the world, and that's where HCA came in.[48]

When Dr. Rifat asked Hill why he wanted to expand into Saudi Arabia, Hill replied that "overseas people, particularly in Europe and the Middle East and Far East, think that the only thing Americans do is produce Coca-Cola and make automobiles. There's a great deal more to our country than that. I don't see why we don't export our expertise in the healthcare area."[49]

With that, Hill sent a team of experts, including Frist Jr., George Mercy, and Vice President Thomas W. Todd, to Riyadh to analyze the hospital. "Our

Above and right: HCA began a management contract with the King Faisal Specialist Hospital in Riyadh, Saudi Arabia, in 1973. The hospital opened in 1975 and offered the latest technologies to enhance patient care.

Below: John Neff and His Excellency Dr. Rifat Alsayed Ali, personal physician to Saudi Arabia's King Faisal, sign a management contract for the new, $75 million hospital being built by King Faisal.

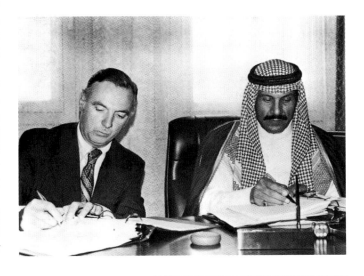

HCA International

IN THE EARLY 1970S, HCA BEGAN TO explore the possibility of international expansion. George Mercy, who had previously worked for an oil company that required him to travel and live in a number of foreign countries, began traveling internationally to look at hospital opportunities, initially in Greece, France, and Spain. Mercy saw HCA's greatest opportunities in developing countries that were member nations of the Organization of Petroleum Exporting Countries (OPEC). These countries had become wealthy from oil exploration and were interested in providing healthcare for their citizens rather than sending them to other countries for healthcare services.

In early 1973, Mercy, Dr. Frist Jr., and Tom Todd, HCA's first vice president of international, traveled to Saudi Arabia at the request of the personal physician to King Faisal. The government of Saudi Arabia was constructing the new $75 million King Faisal Specialist Hospital and research center in Riyadh and was looking for someone to manage it. In the fall of 1973, HCA signed a seven-year contract to manage the Riyadh facility. HCA opened its primary international office in London in 1974 and later opened recruiting offices in the Philippines, Australia, Egypt, Lebanon, and Saudi Arabia. Under the direction of Ron Marston, who would later head HCA International, a school was established in the Philippine Islands to train more than 100 nurses a year to American professional standards and provide the graduates employment in HCA hospitals throughout the world.

Within a couple of years, HCA was faced with a decision about whether to return its Saudi Arabian profits to the United States and pay U.S. income taxes or to reinvest these pretax earnings internationally. Additional opportunities were explored in the Middle East, Europe, Latin America, and Australia. In 1978, under the direction of Bob Crosby, who headed HCA International for several years, the company launched a major expansion program in Australia. HCA committed $45 million for acquisitions of hospitals and construction of new facilities. After a year, HCA owned and operated 10 hospitals in Australia. By this time, it was also managing its second hospital in Saudi Arabia and a hospital in Panama. In 1979 HCA acquired AMICO, a Brazilian health maintenance organization that operated five hospitals and more than 40 clinics and ambulatory centers across Brazil.

In the early 1980s, HCA's international operations expanded to include management of hospitals in India and the Virgin Islands. In 1982 HCA acquired seven hospitals in the United Kingdom and one in Panama. By the end of that year, HCA International owned or managed 32 hospitals in seven countries.

For more than 15 years, HCA's international operations provided growth opportunities for the company and excellent operating returns. It was only during HCA's years as a private company, from 1989 to 1992 (after the leveraged buyout by management), that the company divested its international operations. During this time, the company changed its strategic focus and significantly downsized its operations to include only market-leading hospitals in the United States. Then with the Galen merger in 1993, HCA reentered the international market. In 2003 it had six of the leading private hospitals in London and two in Geneva, Switzerland.

evaluation team came away with the impression that the facility was going to be one of the most outstanding in the world," said Mercy, "that the country was looking for quality care and expertise, and that we had the capabilities, expertise, and desire."[50]

Within months, the three-man management team was negotiating the contract. Then came the 1973–1974 Arab oil crisis. Frist Jr. remembered that while they were in negotiations, the king and his advisors were in the same Geneva hotel "negotiating for Phantom jets and weapons to supply the

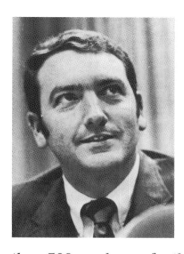

Robert Crosby joined HCA in 1969. He later became a senior vice president and president of HCA International. He retired in 1983.

armament to neutralize the situation in the Middle East."[51]

Over the next two years, HCA recruited and relocated more than 500 employees for the Middle Eastern operation, which had attracted hundreds of applicants from Europe, the United States, and the Middle East. The facility, called by some the "most advanced and sophisticated medical center in the world," opened in 1975.[52] It quickly turned into a medical city complex, encompassing power plants, transportation systems, and housing. "The hospital itself is just one segment of the overall medical community, and we manage the whole medical city," said Crosby.[53]

Operations Decentralize

Expanding as if by centrifugal force, HCA worked hard to manage its phenomenal success. In 1971 it reviewed its operating methods and realigned responsibilities of senior company officials. John Neff became executive vice president and a full-time member of the executive committee. The following year he was named president and chief executive officer of HCA, succeeding John Hill, who became chairman until his retirement in 1977. Frist Jr. was named executive vice president of development, which included all acquisition and construction activities. Bob Brueck took charge of operations for all existing hospitals in his new post as senior vice president.[54]

It was through Brueck's direction that the company reorganized itself in 1973 into nine geographically aligned operating divisions. George Mercy had already been operating HCA's Western Division hospitals, and his work laid the philosophical groundwork for organizing the company on a decentralized,

divisional basis. Mercy's Western Division was thriving under his oversight.[55]

Rather than having to go to the corporate office for key operating decisions, divisions had direct responsibility for their hospitals. Each divisional vice president—along with Bob Brueck and Andrew "Woody" Miller, operations controller, who would later become president of HCA Management Company—made up the company's operations committee. The operations committee met regularly to discuss planning processes, administrative coordination, financial matters, development and implementation of information systems, and movement of human resources.[56]

First Plateau

At its five-year milestone, 1973, Hospital Corporation of America surpassed $200 million in total revenues and $12 million in net income (an 18 percent increase over net income the year before). The company declared its first cash dividend, a six-cent-per-share semiannual distribution. HCA operated 57 hospitals, comprising 8,500 beds, in 13 states.

It was a year of other firsts. Several of the larger hospitals pioneered new procedures. In its first year of operation, North Florida Regional in Gainesville performed more than 900 cardiac catheterizations. Los Robles, near Los Angeles, had a very active open heart surgery unit. University Hospital in Lubbock, Texas, was the site of the nation's first successful artificial ankle joint implantation, in which a prosthetic joint replaced a degenerative arthritic ankle.[57]

Having built more hospitals than any other organization in the world, the company had, during its brief history, acquired vast experience in hospital design, construction, financing, equipping, and staffing. Its accomplishments drew the interest of numerous analysts from Wall Street and investment banking firms. The company enjoyed favorable coverage in such publications as *Forbes,* the *National Observer, Hospital World,* and *Barron's,* and in media in the communities where HCA had a hospital. Ground-breaking ceremonies, ribbon cuttings, and open houses, often attended by large crowds, helped stimulate the local media's interest. More than 15,000 people toured HCA's new Medical Center Hospital in Selma, Alabama, during its grand opening in the summer of 1971.[58]

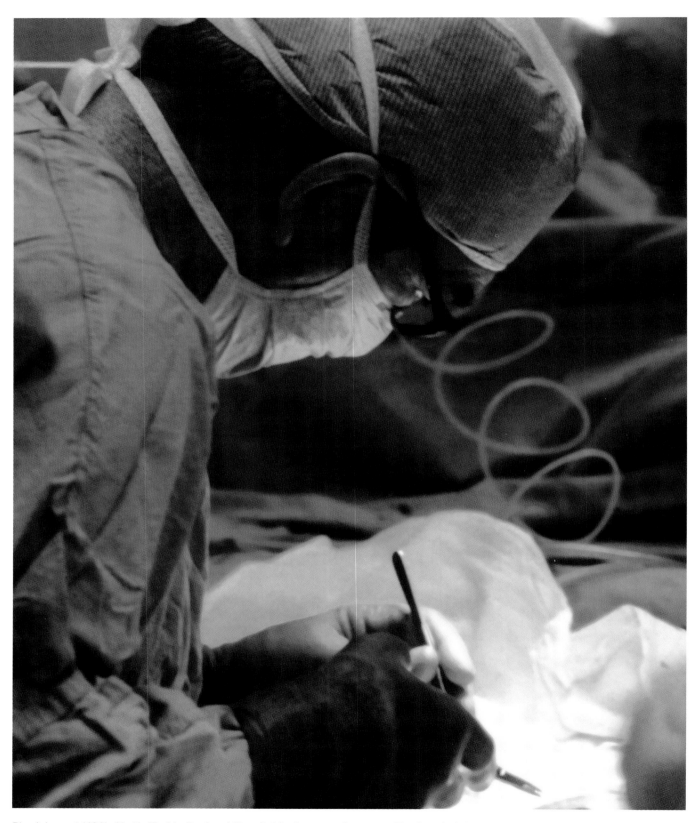

Physicians at HCA's North Florida Regional Hospital in the operating room. The hospital, located in Gainesville, was one of 15 owned by HCA in the state in 1978.

CHAPTER THREE

FORMULA FOR SUCCESS

1974 – 1978

The pioneering efforts of [HCA's founders] and the success HCA has enjoyed during its first decade have encouraged others from the private sector to become more involved in the nation's healthcare delivery system. This, in our opinion, is good for the country and our industry.

—Donald MacNaughton and Thomas Frist Jr., 1978

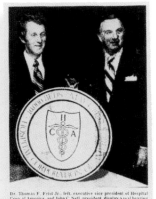

Dr. Thomas F. Frist Jr., left, executive vice president of Hospital Corp. of America, and John C. Neff, president, display a seal bearing the firm's corporate emblem which denotes reaching more than 10,000 beds in operation.

Hospital Corp. Adds Facility, Has 10,000 Beds In Operation

YEARS LATER, JACK MASSEY remarked casually to a reporter that HCA had "exceeded our fondest hopes." Despite the quiet confidence of his crowning years, Massey played many key roles in the company's development.

Some who knew him said he had a gift. Just as the rare individual is born with an ear keenly attuned to music or to the grace and rhythm and power of words, Jack Massey knew how to turn visionary ideas into practical, profitable business plans.

He was also one of the top players of his time when it came to mergers and acquisitions. "He could sit across the negotiating table and appear to hypnotize someone into thinking that it was their deal," said Frist Jr. "Many times, I'd be on an airplane with him, and by the time we landed, the people didn't even know that they'd been hypnotized, and we got the deal we wanted."[1]

Carl George, who began working for HCA in 1969 as assistant treasurer and later became senior vice president of development, remembered a story that illustrated Massey's adeptness at making deals. After a full day of meetings to court lenders, Massey would sometimes invite employees back to his home for cocktails. "We were at Mr. Massey's house, and we were admiring the Persian rug he had. So he started telling a story

about how he had negotiated to buy that rug by bringing three checks with him," George said. "The checks were already made out in three different amounts, and Massey pulled out the lowest check and told the vendor it was all he had to spend. The vendor at first argued that the price was too cheap, but "ultimately, he didn't have to go for the second or third check," said George.[2]

Helen King Cummings, who joined HCA in 1968, when the company acquired Lady Anne Memorial Hospital in Livingston, Tennessee, was appointed HCA's first woman vice president by Massey in 1977. She remembered Massey as a remarkable person. "He had tremendous business ability," she recalled seven years after her retirement in 1995 as vice president of health financing. "He believed in people and wanted to see people achieve tremendous accomplishments in life. He always believed in me, and you don't forget people like that."[3]

In May 1975, HCA's 10,000th bed was put in operation with the opening of a 320-bed facility in Pensacola, Florida. Thomas Frist Jr. (left), executive vice president, and John Neff, president, pose with a company seal that celebrates that milestone.

In one sense, Massey followed the old American pragmatic view of doing well by doing good. Another perspective held that Massey, like generations of businessmen before him, had figured out how to participate in businesses that require the involvement of the largest presence in the U.S. economy: the federal government.

Speaking to stockholders in 1980, another American business legend, Donald MacNaughton, said of the man he succeeded as head of the company, "Any new, fast-growing corporation faces very serious financial problems, and it was Mr. Massey's knowledge and ability and judgment that carried HCA through those rough waters in the early years."[4]

If Massey was the financial backbone of the company, Frist Sr. was the heart and soul. "They were two of the most wonderful people you'd ever meet, both truly southern gentlemen," said

Vic Campbell, who began at the company in 1972 and rose to become senior vice president for investor relations, government relations, and communications. "Jack Massey was a businessman; Dr. Frist Sr. was a humanitarian. They had a great rapport. You didn't want Frist Sr. running the company alone because he'd give it away. And you probably didn't want Jack Massey running the company alone because he was so financially focused. They were just a great blend."[5]

In 1974, Jack Massey (left) assumed the post of chairman of the executive committee after having served as chairman of the board since the company's founding. He poses here with cofounder Thomas Frist Sr. and the certificate of appreciation presented to Massey at the December 1974 board meeting.

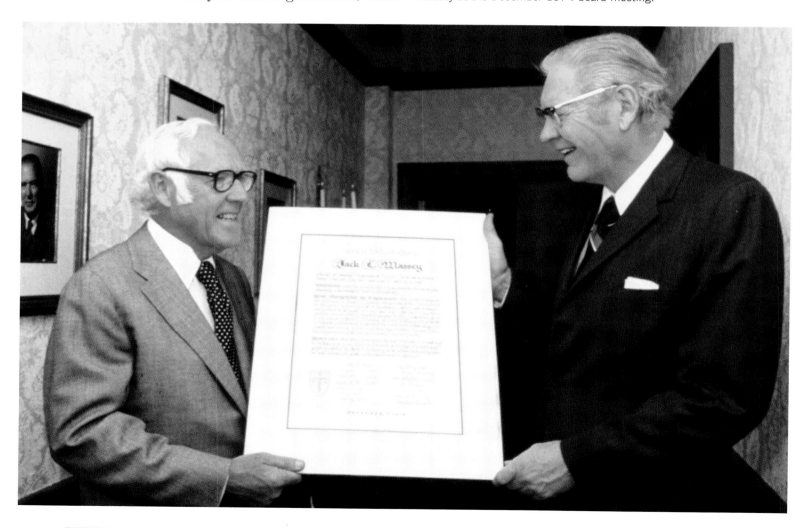

"Doc Frist Sr. was the one everybody at the company would call on for help," said George. "With all his patients, he still had the best bedside manner. He always made you feel like you were the most important person he was talking to or working with at that particular time."[6]

"I'll never forget the first time I met Dr. Frist Sr.," said Jim Fitzgerald, who started in HCA's audit department in 1981 and later became a senior vice president. "I was having lunch in the cafeteria, and he came and sat by me and began talking. He wanted to know about me, my background, my career, my aspirations. I didn't realize this was the founder of the company. And that was one of the things that's always struck me about Tommy and his dad—how they treated people the same whether they were CEO of a *Fortune* 500 company or a brand new auditor, like I was."[7]

Jack Bovender, who later became HCA's president, chairman, and CEO, had a similar impression on first meeting Frist Sr.: "When he came over to talk to you, you were the only person in the room."[8]

It was the Frist family that drove HCA's culture. "The first thing you think of when you think of the name Frist is family," said Campbell. "As employees, we were treated like family."[9]

Helen King Cummings recalled a conversation she had with Frist Sr. that exemplified his personality.

"I appreciate the opportunity to work here at HCA," she told him, "where I'm given responsibility and trust, because I know what it's like to live in poverty."

At that point, Dr. Frist Sr. stopped her. "Helen," he said. "You know what it's like to not have money. You and I have that in common. But we have never known poverty. We have always been exceptionally wealthy in life's true riches, and that's family, friends, honesty, hard work, and making the world a better place."[10]

Dr. Frist Jr. completed HCA's management triumvirate. Like his father, Frist Jr. had a presence about him that made those who came in contact with him want to do their best. He also brought an instinctual decision-making ability to HCA's operations, and his forthright approach and honesty made him an ideal leader, especially in such a people-oriented field as healthcare.

Dr. Frist Sr. touched the lives of many, including Helen King Cummings, who became HCA's first female vice president.

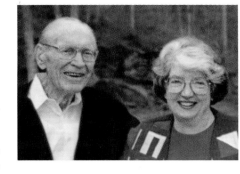

"Tommy Frist Jr. has an incredible ability to look into the future and sort of think, 'You know, if this happens, we should position this way, and if this other thing happens, we should position a different way,'" said Noel Williams, who began with HCA in 1979 and later became senior vice president and chief information officer. "He's a great leader, and he sets an incredible example for all of us. His approach to decision making, the way he balances work and family, his philanthropy. He's just sets a great example."[11]

"I learned this business from Tommy," said Richard Bracken, who joined HCA in 1981 and later became president and chief operating officer. "His way of mentoring was an everyday kind of thing. It was all the little decisions that made a company work, that made people better, and it showed up every day in small ways and large ways. His mentoring was a consistent theme of how to run an organization, how to handle yourself as a person and as a professional, how to have a long view of success."[12]

"Tommy has always been a visionary," said Clayton McWhorter, who joined HCA in 1970 and later became president, chief operating officer, and chairman of Columbia/HCA. "He's a thinker. He's a dreamer. I don't know how many times I've said 'I wish I had thought of that' when he comes up with an idea."[13]

Steve Riven, senior managing director at Nashville's AvondalePartners, was nine years old when he met a young Tommy Frist in camp. The two boys became fast friends. They attended Vanderbilt University together and maintained a lifelong friendship. "When Tommy is your mentor, it doesn't mean he's way up there sending advice down from the mountain top," said Riven. "Tommy's idea of mentoring is friendship.... Tommy pushes his friends the same way he pushes himself. He wants us to succeed. He wants us to win. He wants us to be fully engaged in life."[14]

The First Priority: Patients

According to Massey, the founders were just as amazed as everybody else at the success of their enterprise, and the company found itself struggling to master that success throughout the mid-1970s. HCA developed two tools to guide itself, formal mission and philosophy statements, because the Drs. Frist and Jack Massey believed that it was important to pause and think about what HCA valued and what fundamental principles ought to guide it.

In its mission statement, the company declared that it planned to attain international leadership in the healthcare field while providing superior services and improved standards in the communities where it had facilities.

At the same time, it would "generate measurable benefits" for itself, physicians and other medical staff, employees, investors, "and, most importantly, The Patient." The philosophical platform turned these overarching goals into specific,

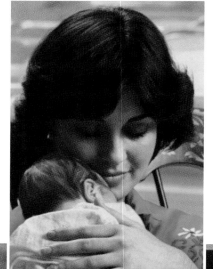

Below left: Renowned for his humanitarian approach to medicine, Dr. Frist Sr. exemplified the company's philosophy of excellence in healthcare.

Below right: The HCA Mission, seen here on a plaque, was first published in the 1974 annual report. As Chairman John Hill reported to HCA shareholders, the mission and philosophy "reflect the original thinking of the founders of our Company, the fundamental concepts which will be its foundation and the moral and ethical guidelines by which it will be managed."

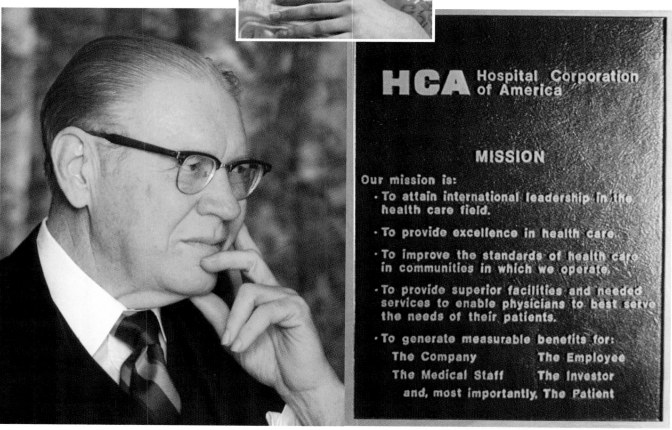

HCA Hospital Corporation of America

MISSION

Our mission is:

- To attain international leadership in the health care field.

- To provide excellence in health care.

- To improve the standards of health care in communities in which we operate.

- To provide superior facilities and needed services to enable physicians to best serve the needs of their patients.

- To generate measurable benefits for:
  The Company   The Employee
  The Medical Staff   The Investor
  and, most importantly, The Patient

tangible objectives. HCA expected high performance from all who worked for and with it. In turn it offered continuing education and information systems. It also encouraged and supported corporate and community citizenship and pledged excellent management underpinned by ethical practices.[15]

This self-examination led to both short-term practical changes and long-term strategizing toward still more growth. But individuals—real people with real pain—were never out of sight, not with Dr. Frist Sr.'s leadership. He had promised in HCA's first annual report that "HCA management [was] dedicated, above all, to warmth and compassion for the patients in its hospitals."[16]

"Don't worry about the bottom line," Frist Sr. used to tell employees. "Put the patient first, and the rest will follow."

In 1974 HCA launched a formal quality assurance program, expanding it to each of its hospitals the next year. It was essentially a management-by-objectives plan for each patient that reported on the patient's health status after treatment and compared it with the expected status.[17]

HCA hospitals continued to become more technologically sophisticated and offered an increased number of specialty services. In previous years, regional medical centers or teaching and research institutions had met this demand, but HCA knew that its patients, their insurance providers, and the general public expected all hospitals to have the "latest and best."

The company also recognized that old-style hospital buildings—sometimes towering boxes or fortress-like institutions—were being succeeded by campus-like settings. Broad vistas under year-round sun in Orlando or long winter nights in Idaho Falls provided comforting settings. Moreover, such sprawling landscapes could accommodate a doctors' office building, diagnostic and laboratory facilities, and an outpatient center alongside the main acute-care facility.[18]

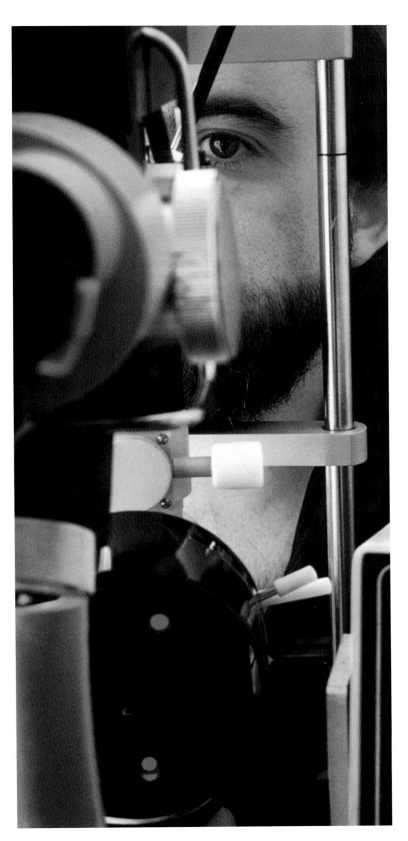

HCA hospitals incorporate state-of-the-art technology, and the company's ability to bring current technology to aging hospitals is one of its hallmarks.

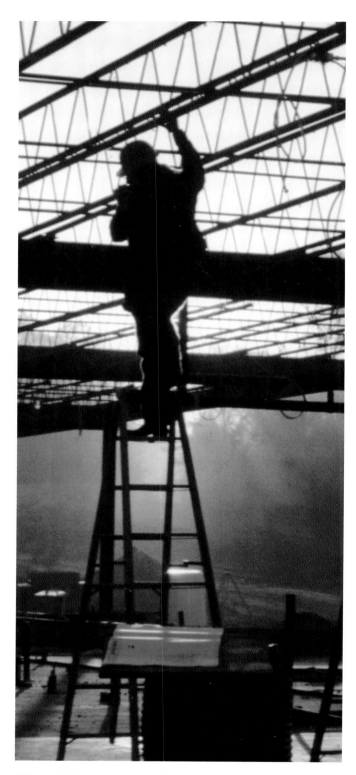

HCA had 16 construction projects under way in 1978, including Nashville's Southern Hills Hospital, a 100-bed facility shown here in the early days of construction.

Setting a Precedent

While continually improving patient care, HCA augmented its infrastructure to maximize efficiencies. From the home office or the regional division, an administrator could get help with accounting, governmental relations, materials management, local tax questions, and many other subjects. But as Frist Jr. pointed out in 1978, "For the most part, our company has been a highly decentralized organization. The key was to bring administrators into our system who could really handle operations on their own while using the tools we provided them."[19]

HCA's customs were catching on, too. Frist Jr. perceived a new role for the private sector in a new day. "You and I were brought up thinking hospitals shouldn't make a profit," he said. "Well, that was in the days when if you needed a $1 million addition, you could raise half through donations. Today that addition might cost $20 million, and you probably still couldn't raise more than $500,000 in donations. We have been the stimulus for a cottage industry to organize itself."[20]

HCA's management contracts continued to improve healthcare and help ailing hospitals. The George W. Hubbard Hospital, on the campus of Meharry Medical College, a mile north of HCA headquarters, became HCA's largest facility under contract in 1978. Meharry was one of two historically black medical schools in the United States, the other being Howard University College of Medicine in Washington, D.C. Hubbard Hospital's deficits had threatened Meharry's existence.[21]

Another success story was Edmond Memorial Hospital just outside Oklahoma City. The institution staggered under the weight of its bonded indebtedness. It had lost national accreditation, and physicians were sending patients elsewhere because of obsolete equipment. A desperate board hired HCA to take over management. By the summer of 1979, the 98-bed hospital had caught up on its bond payments, bought $200,000 worth of the most-needed equipment, and put an almost equal amount in the bank. Its charges rose only about 5 percent during a time when hospital costs generally were rising at three times that pace.[22]

Shifting Roles

After John Neff left HCA in 1976, Jack Massey returned from semiretirement to become president and chief executive officer. At the age of 39, Dr. Frist Jr. was considered too young for the position, but he assumed responsibility for operations of the company as executive vice president and chief operating officer. Then in 1977, Frist Jr. succeeded Massey as president, and Massey became chairman of the board after John Hill retired.[23] Frist Sr. remained vice chairman of the board and chief medical officer.

HCA divided its overseas business into a separate division called HCA International, with senior vice president Robert Crosby as president. Senior vice president Mercy, meanwhile, shifted his responsibility to acquisitions and special projects. And senior vice president R. Clayton McWhorter took over responsibility for domestic operations while senior vice president Dave Williamson headed up domestic development.

McWhorter, who began his career as a hospital pharmacist, joined HCA in 1970 as administrator of the new Palmyra Park Hospital in Albany, Georgia. In 1973 he had been promoted

Inset: Clayton McWhorter joined HCA in 1970 as a hospital administrator. He rose to become president and chief operating officer before departing in 1987 to lead HealthTrust, an HCA spin-off. In 1995, he returned as chairman of Columbia/HCA when it acquired HealthTrust.

Below: In 1977, Thomas Frist Jr. (left) was named president in addition to his duties as chief operating officer. Jack Massey (center), already chief executive officer, was named chairman of the board. Thomas Frist Sr. (right) continued as vice chairman of the board and chief medical officer. That year the company owned or managed 95 hospitals in 24 states plus Panama and Saudi Arabia.

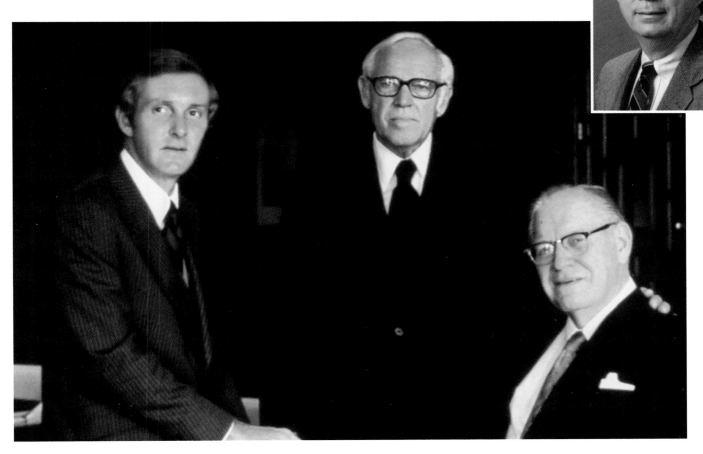

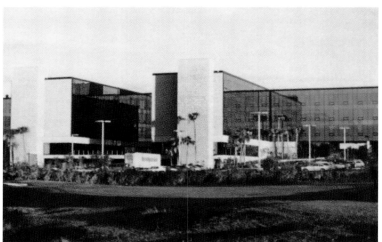

Top: HCA acquired Medical Center Hospital (left) in Largo, Florida, in 1978. Jack Bovender (right), who joined the company in 1975 as an assistant administrator, became the CEO of the hospital. Bovender would later succeed Dr. Frist Jr. as chairman and CEO of HCA.

Below: Carl George, who in 2003 had worked at HCA for 34 years, signs a loan agreement in Australia to finance the company's international equity investment in 1978. At the time, George was CFO of HCA Australia.

to vice president for HCA's hospitals in the southeastern states. One of his major responsibilities in his new position was to maintain the company's decentralized philosophy and local autonomy. "My responsibility is to look at policy from the field point of view, to maintain the balance between field and corporate," he said. "I have to think how corporate decisions are going to be perceived at the division level and the hospital level."[24]

Meanwhile, another key figure in HCA's history was moving through the ranks. Jack Bovender, who by 2002 would be HCA's president, chairman, and CEO, was hired in 1975 as an associate administrator of the new hospital in Pensacola, Florida. The Duke University graduate went on to become division vice president of HCA's Atlantic Division in 1985 and group president of Eastern Group operations in 1987.

HCA's exceptional reputation was based on more than new buildings, technology, and amenities. "It's more than the brick and mortar; it's the people and physicians who make the difference," McWhorter said, borrowing a phrase from Dr. Frist Sr.[25] Having worked his way up from hospital administrator to divisional vice president and then to head of domestic operations, McWhorter knew how important good people and relationships were to HCA's hospitals and to quality care. "Involving physicians in management, getting their input, is invaluable," he said. "And matching up the individual with the position and the responsibilities that go with it is key. You've got to give your administrators the greatest amount of autonomy

and leeway that they can possibly have to operate on a day-to-day basis."[26]

Expanding to a Global Scale

With management of the hospital in Saudi Arabia well under way, HCA was carefully evaluating other international markets. The financial success of the Saudi contract led HCA to a decision: Should it take its Saudi earnings to the United States and pay U.S. income taxes, or should it reinvest pretax earnings overseas? The company decided on the latter.

In 1974 HCA bought Centro Medica Patello in Panama City. Then in 1978 the company expanded into Australia with the purchase of the 196-bed Baulkham Hills Private Hospital in Sydney, Australia. HCA saw Australia as a fertile field

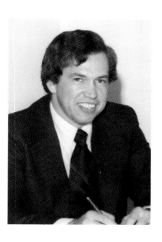

for expansion and a market opportunity similar to that of the United States. "The concept of investor-owned hospitals is in its infancy, and there are no companies such as ours [in Australia]," Dr. Frist Jr. told stockholders. HCA soon acquired three more Australian facilities and announced that negotiations were under way for seven more.

This 1974 graphic illustrates the geographic distribution of the company's holdings. Solid circles represent hospitals in operation, hollow circles are hospitals in operation while being expanded or replaced, solid triangles are new hospitals under construction, and hollow triangles represent HCA-managed hospitals under construction.

Getting Noticed

As HCA and the investor-owned hospital sector grew, the business press took note. In a 1974 survey of the 929 largest public companies in the nation, *Forbes* ranked HCA 29th in five-year revenue growth and 51st in earnings-per-share growth.

HCA placed its 10,000th bed in operation on May 4, 1975. This was a milestone that Jack Massey had once projected wouldn't occur for three more years. HCA had other milestones to celebrate in 1975. No company had ever operated at the capacity HCA had achieved, and it became the first hospital management company to make a public offering of bonds.[27]

But even with all of the attention HCA was receiving, and even though analysts followed the

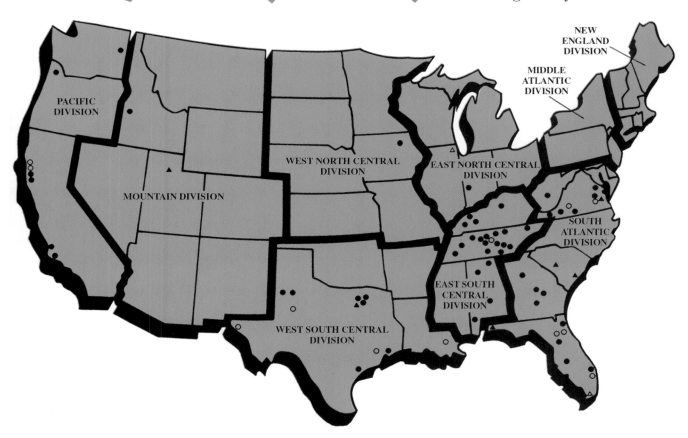

Mexico City

Nashville

Panama City

Riyadh

NEW ENGLAND DIVISION

MIDDLE ATLANTIC DIVISION

PACIFIC DIVISION

WEST NORTH CENTRAL DIVISION

EAST NORTH CENTRAL DIVISION

MOUNTAIN DIVISION

SOUTH ATLANTIC DIVISION

EAST SOUTH CENTRAL DIVISION

WEST SOUTH CENTRAL DIVISION

Members of HCA's board of directors gathered for this group photograph at Nashville's Parthenon in Centennial Park in October 1978. Standing in front: Donald MacNaughton (left) and Winfield Dunn. Seated, from left: Carl Reichardt, Jack Massey, Thomas Frist Sr., John Hill, Thomas Frist Jr., and Millard Bartels. Standing in rear, from left: Robert Brueck, George Alexander, C. George Mercy, David Williamson, Richard Perkins, Thomas Johns, and Max Diamond. Not pictured: Robert Anderson, John deButts, and William Weaver.

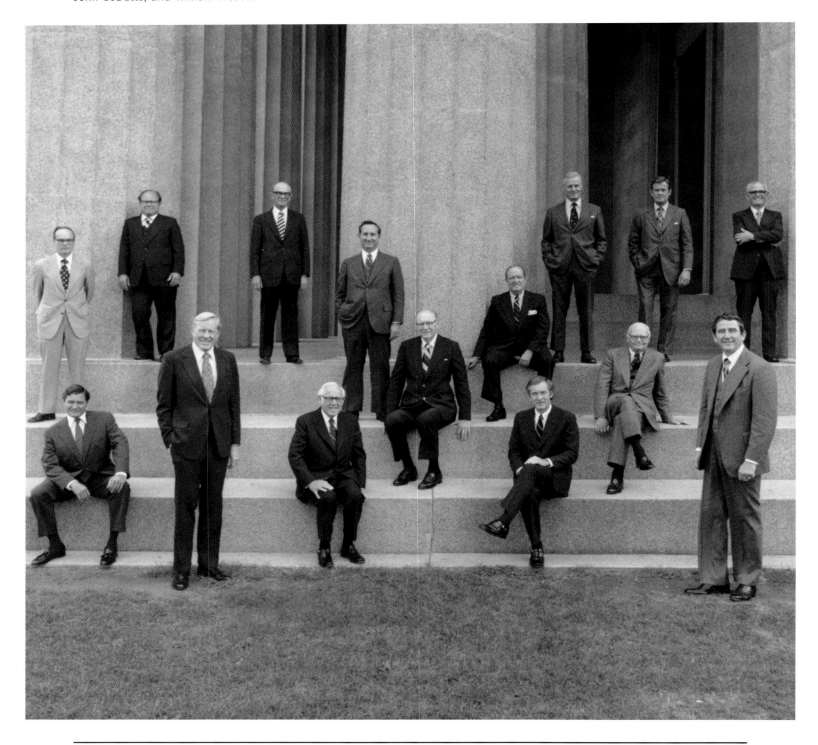

drug and hospital supply industries, Wall Street had not yet recognized hospital management companies as an industry sector. Under Massey's tutelage, Vic Campbell made frequent trips to New York to create an awareness in the investment community that Wall Street should commit analyst resources to cover hospital management as an industry sector. Campbell talked about HCA's story and the opportunities within the industry. He laid out HCA's accomplishments and explained how they had been largely ignored by investors.

John Hindelong, managing director at Donaldson, Lufkin & Jenrette (later Credit Suisse), was one of the first analysts who recognized HCA as the leader in a new industry. "I made a pretty significant bet on HCA and on the industry," Hindelong said more than 20 years later. "Between Vic Campbell and Tommy Frist and the management team at HCA, I was convinced that this company was going to do very well." Though Hindelong followed the entire sector, which included AMI, NME, Humana, and Hospital Affiliates, HCA was the first hospital management company stock that he officially recommended.[28]

Still, it wasn't until 1980 that *Institutional Investor (II)* magazine—after hearing from Campbell for three years—introduced hospital management as an industry. "*II* finally told me that if I promised not to come back next year, they would do it," Campbell said. "That opened the door. From then on, analysts competed for the top spot in the hospital industry just as they had competed in other industries."[29]

Not surprisingly, the magazine cited Hindelong as the first-place hospital management analyst that year—and for many future years—which meant institutional investors recognized him as the most knowledgeable source of information and investment guidance for that industry.

Analyst coverage of HCA grew to include all major national investment firms as well as many regional brokerage firms. Hospital analysts recognized by *Institutional Investor* and others over the years include Paul Becker, Tom McGinnis, Carl Sherman, Ken Abramowitz, Joyce Albers, Geoffrey Harris, Margo Vignola, Todd Richter, Roberta Walter, A. J. Rice, Deborah Lawson, Lori Price, Adam Feinstein, Andrew Bach, and Ken Weakley.

A New Leader

On April 21, 1978, some 700 shareholders convened for the annual meeting at Opryland Hotel at Nashville's famed Opryland theme park. Jack Massey remarked on the astonishing turnout for HCA's 10-year anniversary and added some historical perspective.

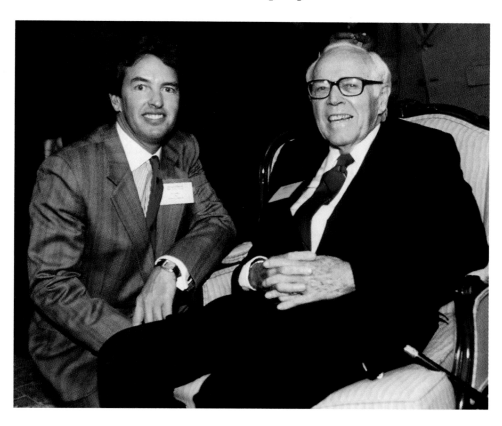

Vic Campbell (left), who in 2003 had been with HCA for 31 years, with his mentor, Jack Massey. In the mid-1970s, Massey taught Campbell how to work with Wall Street.

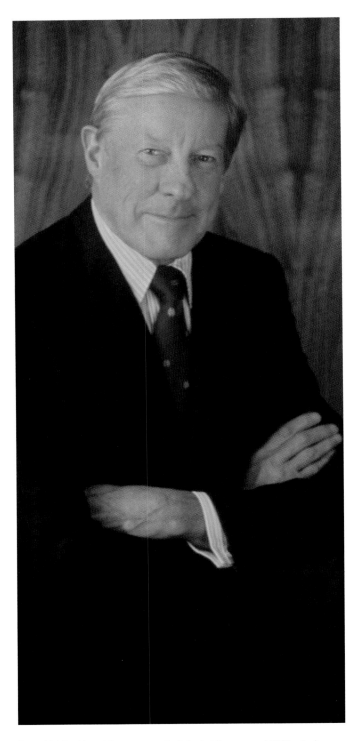

Donald MacNaughton succeeded Jack Massey as HCA's chairman and chief executive officer on October 1, 1978. In this 10th-anniversary year, HCA's revenues reached $797 million, and net income was $42 million. *(Photograph by Wayne Buchanan, Dynamic Media, Inc.)*

We have already reached our goal, set 10 years ago, of operating 100 hospitals by the end of our first 10 years. There was then no hospital management industry as we know it today . . . and there are now more than 30 companies managing almost 600 American hospitals. . . . We really started something back in 1968![30]

Dr. Frist Jr. cast the company's first years in slightly different terms. Historians of HCA recognized his ability to organize the company's story into interesting patterns of insight, interpretation, and understanding—as if he were standing aside from it instead of being its longest full-time employee and the visionary responsible for much of its success. In 1978 he commented particularly on the increasing role of the federal government. "Every time [the federal government] has taken some action in the hospital sector, it has created new opportunities for us," he observed. "We must, however, recognize them and capitalize on them."[31]

When the board convened that summer, it elected Donald S. MacNaughton chairman and chief executive officer, succeeding Jack Massey, who remained chairman of the company's executive committee. Massey had come back into active management at HCA in 1976 to help groom Frist Jr. to someday be CEO. The board began searching for someone who could continue mentoring Frist Jr. Don MacNaughton was clearly the right man for the job.

MacNaughton had recently retired as chairman and CEO of Prudential Insurance Company of America, the largest insurance company in the world. He had led Prudential through a period of growth without parallel in the industry, diversifying its lines, restructuring its management, and expanding its operations overseas.[32]

Years later, MacNaughton told how HCA managed to recruit him. While vacationing in Hawaii before his retirement, he had discovered boredom. "I think I played golf four days in a row," he said, "and at the end of the fourth day, I walked off the course. I was so bored with it. Then when I retired from Prudential, I held a press conference to introduce my successor. I also made it clear that I wanted to continue to work. In other words, I used the press conference, among other things, as an opportunity to look for a job."[33]

Frist Jr. remembered what happened next. "Mr. MacNaughton's retirement announcement from Prudential appeared in the *Wall Street Journal*, and the board said, 'Let's go get this man to be the chairman and CEO of HCA!' "[34]

Frist Jr. acknowledged that recruiting MacNaughton was a long shot. Indeed, the former Prudential CEO received some 24 offers over the next few months and finally weeded them down to four or five.

"One that never went away was HCA," MacNaughton said. "I put that one on the back burner, primarily because it didn't fit my geographic description of a job, but it stayed on the list because I had developed a great interest in the healthcare delivery system. And it also stayed on the list because the people from Nashville were very persuasive."[35]

"The board went after him," said Frist Jr. "Dad and the others did a great job talking him into coming."[36]

Dr. Frist Sr. described MacNaughton as "a very sensitive, intelligent, experienced man with great wisdom. . . . With his coming to this company we'll have a greater future to grow and serve the human race than we had the opportunity to do in the past."[37]

Indeed, under MacNaughton's leadership, HCA moved from its entrepreneurial stage into a more global, blue-chip company, though nearly 10 years later, MacNaughton still characterized the company as entrepreneurial. "He saw the big picture," said Frist Jr. "He changed the character of the company. . . . He helped HCA become larger, better known, better respected, and helped HCA find its place in the history of healthcare."[38]

And just as Dr. Frist Sr. and HCA's board had intended, MacNaughton helped groom Frist Jr. to one day become HCA's top leader. "MacNaughton was a tremendous influence on Tommy," said Clayton McWhorter. "Tommy was the visionary, the entrepreneur, and he could move pretty fast sometimes. But MacNaughton was kind of his guiding hand. He was firm, very firm, and he was a real stabilizer."[39]

After only 10 years, HCA operated the world's leading network of hospitals, with more than 120 facilities housing 18,000 beds in 25 states and four foreign countries. It held management contracts with 30 hospitals, which operated an additional 4,500 beds.[40]

And from its founding through its first decade, the company had never experienced a quarter, much less a year, in which revenues and earnings did not increase substantially.

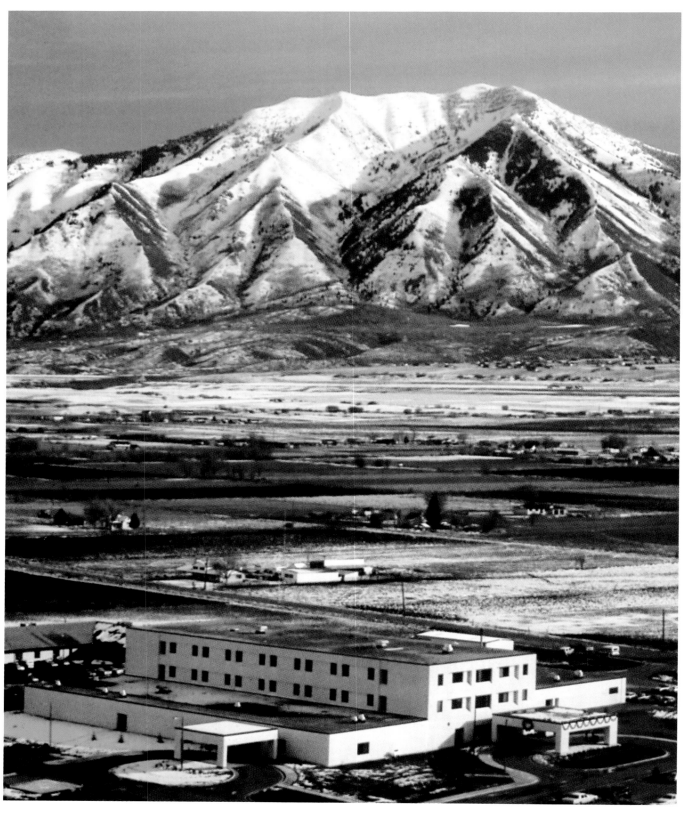

The Rocky Mountains form a majestic backdrop for Mountain View Hospital in Payson, Utah, built by HCA in 1980. The hospital was located in the county with the highest birth rate in the nation.

CHAPTER FOUR

AWESOME GROWTH

1979–1985

We have been strongly impressed by HCA's philosophy, which recognizes that its greatest assets are its employees.

—Harry Neer, president of Presbyterian Hospital, Oklahoma City, 1984

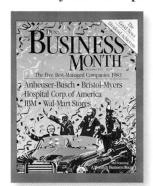

HCA SOARED TO NEW HEIGHTS in the late 1970s and early 1980s. MacNaughton helped the company's management team achieve its true potential by challenging them to think bigger and to broaden their view of the world. Under his firm hand, the company amplified its system of structured management, which better suited the large company that HCA had become.[1]

MacNaughton also fostered the caring work environment that had become HCA's trademark. Helen King Cummings remembered being called into the chairman's office. "And you don't take that lightly when you're called into Mr. MacNaughton's office," she said.

But MacNaughton hadn't summoned her to reprimand her; rather, he was concerned because he hadn't seen her usual smile in a few days.

Stunned that HCA's chairman and CEO would take such a personal interest in her well-being, Cummings told him she was concerned about the recent national issues that were affecting HCA.

MacNaughton reflected for a moment, then said, "Remember, this too shall pass. A year from now, you'll have a different issue that will seem almost as consuming as the one you're going through right now. But it will change. Just remember to keep the current situation in the proper perspective. This is only temporary."

Hearing those words of encouragement, Cummings couldn't help but smile.[2]

MacNaughton also helped build an eminent board of directors comprising some of the nation's top business leaders who, together, represented a world of experience. Frist Jr. described the board as encompassing "not only successful businessmen, but individuals who have achieved every business success one could want. They are among a handful of individuals who have addressed major societal issues and really changed the country outside of their own industry. They were the ones that our country looked to as leaders."[3]

Astronaut Frank Borman, chairman, president, and CEO of Eastern Air Lines and later chairman and CEO of Patlex Corporation, joined HCA's board in 1980, as did Owen Butler, chairman of Procter & Gamble. Irving Shapiro, retired chairman and CEO of DuPont, who sat on the boards of Boeing, IBM, and Citicorp and Citibank, among others, joined HCA's board in 1981. Frank Cary, former chairman and CEO of IBM and a director of J. P. Morgan, PepsiCo, Texaco, and other esteemed companies, became an HCA director in 1982. Donald Seibert, former chairman and CEO of J. C. Penney and a director of Citicorp and Citibank, began serving on HCA's board in 1985.

Dun's Business Month magazine named HCA one of the nation's "Five Best-Managed Companies" in 1982.

Clifton Garvin, chairman and CEO of Exxon and a director of Citicorp and Citibank, Johnson & Johnson, J. C. Penney, PepsiCo, and TRW, came on HCA's board in 1986, as did Martin Feldstein, professor of economics at Harvard, president and CEO of the National Bureau of Economic Research, and former chairman of President Reagan's Council

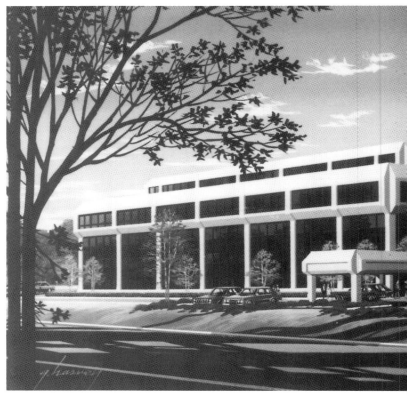

Right: This rendering by Gresham and Smith Architects shows the newly expanded headquarters of HCA in Nashville. Completed in December 1981, the building was twice as large as the old headquarters office.

Below: From its earliest days, HCA was well appreciated in its hometown, Nashville. In April 1979, Nashville and Opryland Hotel honored HCA with an exhibit titled "Salute to HCA." Pictured from left are Winfield Dunn, senior vice president of public affairs; Thomas Frist Jr., president and chief operating officer; Eddie Jones, executive director of the Chamber of Commerce; Mike Diamond, Opryland Hotel; David Williamson, HCA executive vice president; Rudy Caduff, Opryland Hotel; and Jack Vaughn, Opryland Hotel.

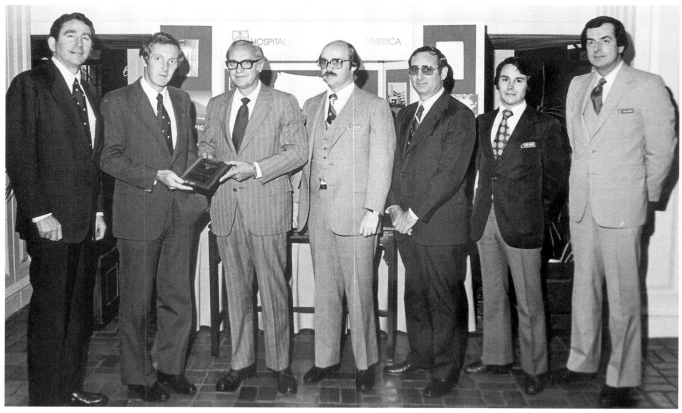

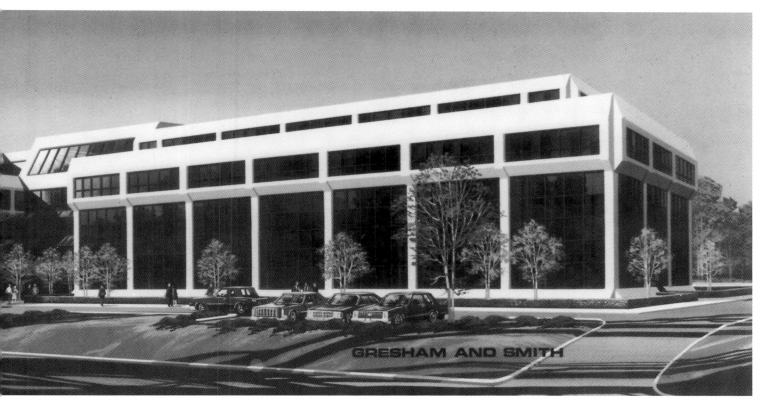

GRESHAM AND SMITH

of Economic Advisors. These esteemed business minds joined Robert Anderson, chairman and CEO of Rockwell International, who had sat on HCA's board since 1971, and Carl Reichardt, chairman and CEO of Wells Fargo and a director of Ford Motor Company, who had joined HCA's board in 1972.

MacNaughton's mere presence helped the company grow. As Frist Jr. pointed out in 1987, "With his name, his image, and the comfort level that people had with his being chairman and CEO, we were able to make acquisitions that we maybe couldn't have made otherwise."[4]

Acquisitions

Under MacNaughton's and Frist Jr.'s leadership, the company went into acquisition mode. "This is a capital intensive industry, and we were in an era of double-digit inflation," Frist Jr. recalled. "So I thought, how do we take advantage of that? If you have your cost fixed on your capital side in a capital-intensive industry, then your revenues are going to go up a lot faster. So with that in mind, we started looking for acquisitions of investor-owned hospital systems and leading not-for-profit hospitals."[5]

In 1980, the company added 25 U.S. hospitals to its network, the largest number of hospitals acquired by HCA in a single year. Six of these came from buying General Health Services, a public company based in California, for $96 million. The company also purchased General Care, based in Nashville, for $78 million. General Care, which owned eight hospitals when HCA acquired it, had begun as a nursing home company but changed into a hospital company. General Care grew mainly by soliciting doctors to become partnership owners in its local hospitals, a practice that HCA frowned upon as a potential conflict of interest for physicians referring patients to facilities they co-owned. Years later, Frist Jr. would unwind physician ownership in hospitals acquired by HCA.[6]

In 1981, HCA bought four hospitals from Health Care Corporation for $30 million and made its biggest acquisition yet when it purchased Hospital Affiliates International (HAI), then a wholly owned subsidiary of INA Corporation, for $650 million. HAI, also based in Nashville, had been founded in 1968, a few months before HCA went public, by two former physician-owners of Park View. HAI spent its early years managing hospitals for other owners before moving into ownership. In 1977, HAI sold itself to INA Corporation, an insurance company based in Philadelphia. HCA had been interested in buying HAI, but the Nashville rivalry of HCA and HAI precluded the sale. Later, however, INA, which was removed from local Nashville politics, sold its HAI subsidiary to HCA. At the time, HAI owned 55 hospitals (including 19 psychiatric facilities) and managed another 78 hospitals.

MacNaughton was instrumental in the purchase of HAI, "primarily because of personal knowledge of the players at INA," said Clayton McWhorter, who became the company's chief operating officer in 1983. "He gave our board of directors a comfort level in doing a deal of that magnitude."[7]

HAI's hospitals not only complemented HCA's existing markets; they gave HCA a leadership position in the psychiatric field and, in the words of Frist Jr., "really put us in the driver's seat in the management contract business."[8] (By the time HCA sold its management contract segment in 1989, it managed more than 200 hospitals.)

Earnings per share showed healthy growth. The acquisition of HAI produced a vast gain in revenues. And with the three other public hospital companies HCA bought in 1980 and 1981, the size of the company nearly doubled. HCA's revenues in 1982 reached nearly $3 billion.[9]

Though HCA's debt had mounted to 65 percent of capitalization in early 1982 to finance acquisitions and capital investments, by the end of the year its debt had slimmed to 57 percent of capitalization, and it continued to ratchet downward through the mid-1980s.[10]

Strengthening the Network

In 1983 HCA invested about $650 million in acquisition and construction, acquiring four hospitals, finishing construction on 18 others, and completing 42 expansions of beds and services. It also added 38 management contracts in 1983 and another 34 in 1984, bringing HCA Management Company's total number of managed hospitals to 187. Internationally, HCA constructed four more hospitals in the United Kingdom and one in Brazil and acquired a hospital in Australia. By the end of 1984, HCA International owned and operated 25 hospitals and managed six others.[11] In 1985 HCA

added 17 general hospitals, 13 psychiatric hospitals, and 27 domestic management contracts, plus two management contracts in Canada.[12]

By the mid-1980s, HCA had gained a high level of credibility in the industry. Recent trends in healthcare led not-for-profit hospitals to seek relationships with HCA, which could provide professional management and much-needed capital. These affiliations were a significant step in HCA's growth, for never before had HCA been able to acquire such preeminent hospitals.

After studying the current trends in healthcare and how those changes were likely to shape the future of the country's healthcare delivery system, the not-for-profit Wesley Medical Center in Wichita, Kansas, approached HCA in 1984. A. B. Davis Jr., president and CEO of Wesley Corporation and Wesley Medical Center, described HCA as "a company recognized worldwide for its high quality, patient-oriented care." With 760 beds, Wesley Medical Center became the largest of HCA's hospitals and was a major diagnostic, therapeutic, and teaching referral center for south central Kansas.[13] It was renowned for its neonatal intensive care unit. By the turn of the century, more than half the babies born in Kansas each year were born at Wesley.

HCA acquired another outstanding not-for-profit in 1984, Oklahoma City's 407-bed Presbyterian Hospital. Its operations included several subcenters, among them the Cancer Institute and the Bob Hope Center for Eye Surgery; the largest remote cardiac monitoring system in the country; a network of eight hospitals throughout Oklahoma; and consulting, clinical, and other support services to more than 50 clinics and hospitals. Presbyterian Hospital chose to affiliate with HCA because HCA shared Presbyterian's basic beliefs. "We have been strongly impressed by HCA's philosophy, which recognizes that its greatest assets are its employees," said Harry Neer, president of Presbyterian Hospital. "We share with HCA the commitment to work in close alliance with physicians, resulting in

Opposite: In 1984 HCA acquired the 760-bed Wesley Medical Center in Wichita, Kansas. Known for forward thinking, Wesley had established Life Watch, an air ambulance service, in 1974.

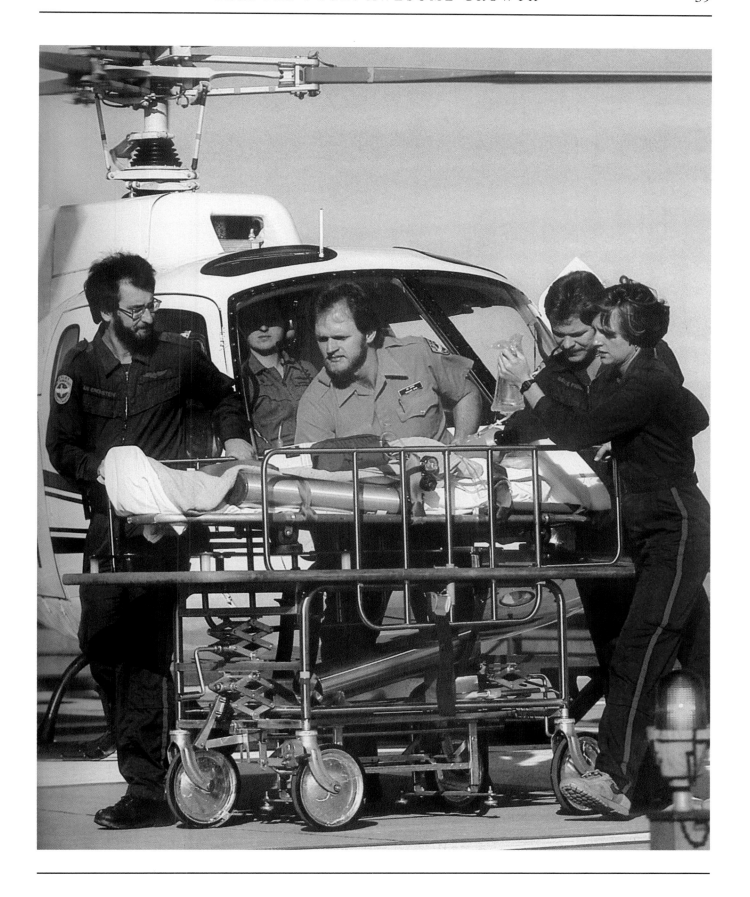

the highest quality of healthcare for the community."[14] (In 1998, HCA would expand its Oklahoma City presence by acquiring University Hospital and Children's Hospital of Oklahoma.)

In 1985, HCA formed a joint venture with the not-for-profit Lovelace Foundation to own 80 percent of a new entity, Lovelace Medical Center, Inc., in Albuquerque, New Mexico. The medical center was a major teaching center affiliated with the University of New Mexico School of Medicine and Allied Health Sciences Center. The joint venture included five affiliated clinics, outpatient services, and the Lovelace Health Plan, an HMO.[15]

Other new ventures enlarged HCA's original vision and strengthened its network of regional healthcare systems. In 1983, HCA entered a management contract with Bascom Palmer Eye Institute at the University of Miami, its first such undertaking at a teaching center. Two other medical schools, the Research Medical Center of Kansas City and Vanderbilt University, built psychiatric facilities jointly with the company. Other managerial and consultative affiliations with academic institutions soon followed, including management of the teaching hospital of the University of Mississippi Medical Center in Jackson. A 1985 agreement with Brigham and Women's Hospital of Boston to exchange educational purchasing services also helped strengthen HCA's network of regional healthcare systems.[16]

Left: In 1985 HCA partnered with the Lovelace Foundation to own 80 percent of Lovelace Medical Center in Albuquerque, New Mexico. Lovelace included five affiliated clinics, outpatient services, and the Lovelace Health Plan, a 50,000-member HMO.

Right: In 1985, the highly respected Scripps Clinic and Research Foundation leased its Green Hospital to HCA.

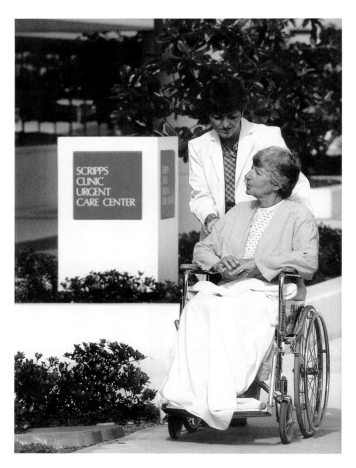

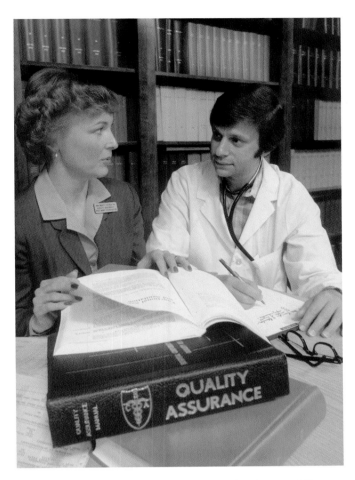

Above and right: HCA hospitals are committed to providing excellent healthcare. The company's formal quality assurance program helps ensure this by measuring the quality of patient care against predetermined standards.

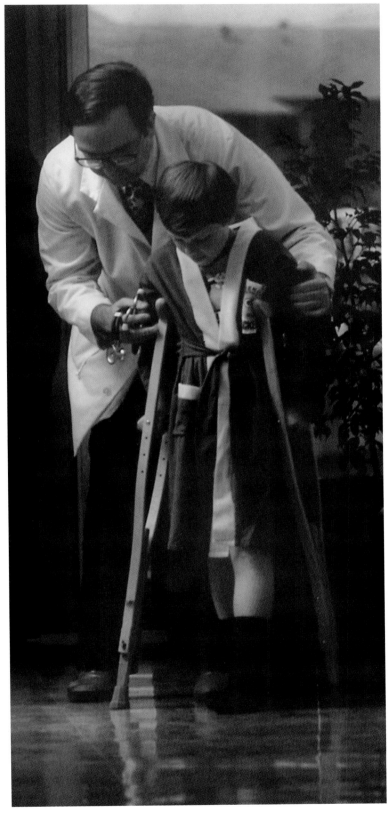

Also in 1985, the not-for-profit Scripps Clinic and Research Foundation in La Jolla, California, began leasing its Green Hospital to HCA, allowing Scripps and its Medical Group to become one of HCA's major worldwide referral centers. "HCA's broader access to capital will put Scripps in an excellent position to add to the capacity and service capabilities of Green Hospital," said Dave Williamson.[17]

At the same time, no one could doubt that HCA was still master of its fundamental business. It built a 100-bed hospital in Tucson, Arizona, in 37 weeks. Its Saudi Arabian subsidiary opened and staffed an $800 million military hospital in 90 days![18]

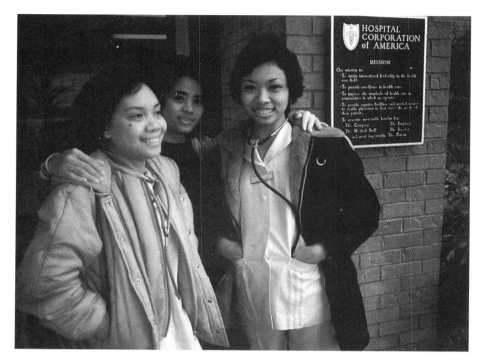

Above: Evangeline Bernardino (right), one of 22 Filipino nurses who came to HCA's Lea Regional Hospital in Hobbs, New Mexico, received training as part of an international medical exchange.

Right: A visitor checks in at the reception area of the Assistencia Medica a Industria e Comercio (AMICO), a wholly owned affiliate of HCA in Brazil. In 1980, AMICO, one of the largest HMOs in Brazil, employed 780 doctors, 680 nurses, and 1,440 other healthcare personnel. It operated five hospitals and 42 ambulatory centers.

To Diversify or Not to Diversify

HCA's board recognized that medical-surgical hospitals would always be an excellent business but that growth through acquisitions might eventually slow due to antitrust considerations and the fact that most hospitals would remain not-for-profit, especially in the Northeast. Therefore, the company, with its concentration of assets in Sunbelt states, decided to carefully test a strategy of diversifying into health-related areas.

The company's old entrepreneurial zest showed in its attempts to find, found, or create these new pockets for investment and to anticipate trends in the industry. It made substantial acquisitions in psychiatric hospitals, becoming the largest private operator of such facilities, with 40 in operation by 1986. It became involved in clinical laboratories, ambulance companies, freestanding primary care centers, and AMICO, a health maintenance organization in Brazil. It also acquired a 17 percent equity position in Beverly Enterprises, the nation's largest nursing home operator, for the purpose of monitoring "developments in geriatric care." By 1985, however, Dr. Frist Jr. had determined that the nursing home business was too different from the hospital business and didn't make long-term strategic sense for HCA, so HCA divested its position.[19] From an investment standpoint, Frist Jr.'s timing was superb; HCA got out of the nursing home business at its peak.

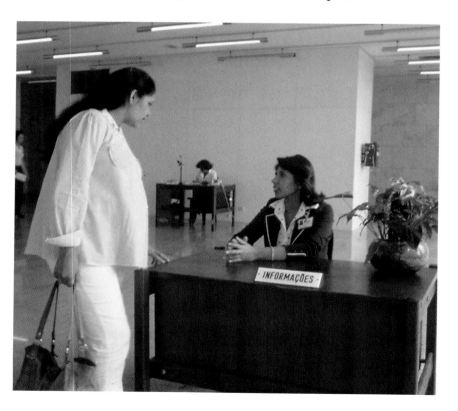

In perhaps the most forward-looking development, company hospitals strengthened their emphasis on outpatient services. Physical therapy and chemotherapy were among these early offerings, but ambulatory surgery and walk-in centers for psychiatric care and drug abuse soon followed.

Market studies showed that women were becoming major purchasers of health services and typically made most health decisions for their families. A number of HCA hospitals established women's centers, where obstetrics, urological and gynecological services, and reconstructive and plastic surgery could be addressed in one highly specialized setting.[20]

Still another opportunity was America's aging population. Forty company hospitals offered a Seniority Program, a package of benefits "designed to build familiarity and trust between the hospital and the community." An adult congregate living facility on HCA's Largo, Florida, campus provided nursing and medical services for patients discharged from the hospital but unable to return home.[21] The plan harkened back to the early days of Park View Hospital in Nashville.

In 1985 HCA sought HMO licenses in 15 states to set up companies that monitored the costs and utilization of health services by their members. Increasingly, academicians and investors were promoting the idea that hospitals should integrate with HMOs as a way to move patients into vacant hospital beds.[22]

HCA also procured insurance licenses in 34 states through the purchase of New Century Life Insurance Company, a subsidiary of E. F. Hutton. HCA's plan was to develop a variety of health insurance products under the leadership of longtime HCA executive Joe Hutts Jr., who was named president of HCA Health Plans. These products ultimately included a national health benefits program intended to be linked to its hospitals and physicians as well as HMOs and preferred provider organizations (PPOs) that it owned or hoped to acquire. The Hill-Richards Company, an insurance claims processing firm that handled more than 300,000 forms in 1984, was added to the HCA quiver as well, and operations were opened in Florida, Louisiana, Tennessee, and Virginia. In another business venture, HCA bought a 20 percent interest in CyCare,

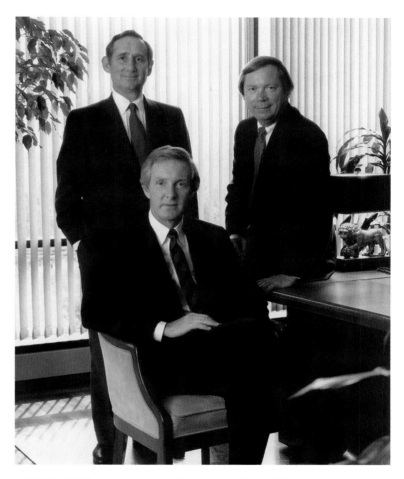

In 1984, HCA's top management team consisted of Thomas Frist Jr. (seated), president and CEO; David Williamson (left), executive vice president of development; and Clayton McWhorter (right), executive vice president of operations.

the nation's leading provider of computer services and systems to physicians and ambulatory care centers. It also formed HCA Physician Services Company in 1985 to provide services to physicians and to strengthen physician relations.[23]

The company's most daring venture was an attempt to acquire American Hospital Supply (AHS), which manufactured and distributed hospital and laboratory supplies as well as instruments and surgical equipment. Merger plans with the Evanston, Illinois, company were announced in March 1985, and it was to be the crown jewel in the "vertically integrated" HCA. The $6.6 billion merger would be the fourth largest in American

FOUNDATIONS FOR GIVING

CHARTERED ON APRIL 19, 1982, THE HCA Foundation was created to fund philanthropic contributions to medical education, the arts, and community service. It was the brainchild of Dr. Frist Jr., who wanted to provide substance and structure to the company's existing philanthropic efforts. He also wanted to develop a vehicle that could develop assets based on HCA's growth.

"The Foundation received a long-term option on a million shares of HCA, and this was something that no one had ever done before," said Pete Bird, executive director and CEO of the Frist Foundation, an offshoot of the HCA Foundation.[1]

At first the option didn't hold a lot of value, so in its early years, the Foundation operated on a pass-through basis: Once a year HCA donated funds to the Foundation based on its profit. The Foundation then dispersed that money to nonprofit organizations.

In 1985 HCA realized a large, one-time gain, so it gave the Foundation $25 million, which covered its donations for the next several years. Then in 1989, when HCA went private, the Foundation was obliged to cash in its stock option. "That gave us about $60 million," said Bird, "which was in turn invested and reinvested and reinvested so that [in 2002] we have about $185 million in assets."[2]

When HCA merged with Columbia in 1994, the Foundation became independent of HCA. Then in 1997, it changed its name to the Frist Foundation. The Frist Foundation name underscored its role as an independent philanthropic organization that served the greater Nashville community while at the same time honoring Dr. Thomas Frist Sr. and Dr. Thomas Frist Jr.

"Our general mission is to invest in the infrastructure of nonprofit organizations to make them stronger and better positioned to serve the community," said Bird.[3]

The Frist Foundation awards about 350 grants a year. A grant to Nashville's Second Harvest Food Bank, for example, helped build a new food warehouse. Another grant helped build three new facilities in Nashville for senior citizens. The Frist Foundation also gives a large grant each year to Junior Achievement and offers significant support to the Special Olympics of Tennessee. Its largest project was the Frist Center for the Visual Arts, a museum arts center in downtown Nashville, which opened in the spring of 2001. The Frist Center

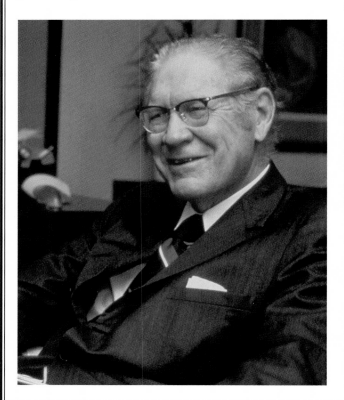

Left: The Frist Foundation is named after Dr. Frist Sr. (pictured), HCA's chief medical director, and his son Dr. Thomas Frist Jr.

Opposite: The Frist Center for the Visual Arts, in Nashville, offers changing exhibits, lecture programs, and special activities. It was funded by the Frist Foundation and Dr. Frist Jr. *(Photo by Timothy Hursley, courtesy of the Frist Center for the Visual Arts.)*

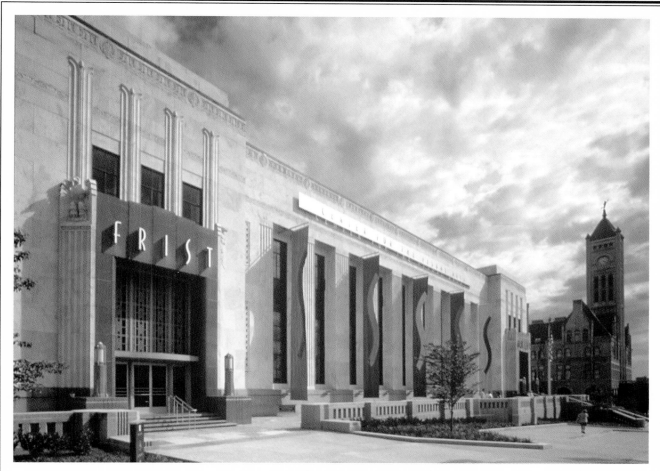

was created in a partnership with the city; the Frist Foundation and Dr. Frist Jr. together donated about $25 million, and the city provided about $20 million. In addition, the Frist Foundation funded the Country Music Hall of Fame and the main library in Nashville and donates to the United Way of Nashville and the Center for Non-Profit Management, which was created by the Frist Foundation to provide training and consulting to nonprofit groups.

Meanwhile, Columbia had acquired its own foundation after it acquired Galen Health Care in 1993. It was later renamed the HCA Foundation and given stock options in HCA, operating as the company's philanthropic arm. Its mission is to promote health and well-being and to support childhood and youth development in middle Tennessee. In partnership with

its employees, it provides leadership, service, and financial support to nonprofit organizations that meet local needs. Every fall, for example, more than 500 HCA employees volunteer for local United Way agencies such as the McNeilly Center for Children and the YWCA Domestic Violence Center. Employees also contribute to the Salvation Army Angel Tree program each year. During the holiday season, trees in the lobbies of HCA headquarters are decorated with angels that bear the name of a child or senior citizen in need. Employees adopt an angel and bring in gifts.[4]

Since 1998, the HCA Foundation has contributed more than $10 million in grants to more than 200 agencies and organizations in Middle Tennessee, focusing on those organizations that promote health and well being, childhood and youth development, and quality of life.[5]

corporate history and the largest outside the oil industry. It would also give HCA a guarantee of supplies at the best price.

The announcement of the pact touched off bitter complaints from other hospitals and hospital chains, which claimed that American Hospital Supply would no longer serve them once in the camp of a competitor. American Medical International in Beverly Hills, California, said it would rebid all its contracts (worth $20 million) with AHS. Atlanta's Shared Services for Southern Hospitals, which represented 174 facilities, made a similar move. AHS's largest customer, Voluntary Hospitals of America in Irving, Texas, established its own supply distribution company, slicing deeply into its $100 million worth of business with the Illinois firm.[24]

Wall Street, generally speaking, did not think much of the idea either. The day after the merger announcement, HCA stock dropped $2.63 a share, or nearly 6 percent, while AHS's fell $3, or 8 percent.[25]

Karl D. Bays (left) of American Hospital Supply and HCA's Thomas Frist Jr. had been working on plans to merge their companies since 1976, but those plans fell apart in 1985 when Baxter Travenol Laboratories stepped in with a higher bid for American Hospital Supply.

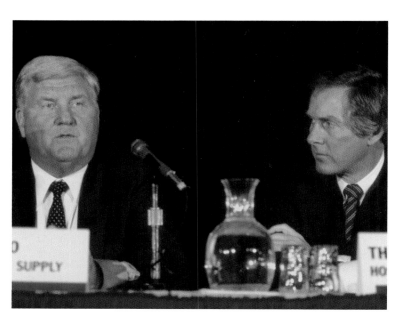

In late summer the merger was challenged by Baxter Travenol Laboratories, AHS's primary competitor and neighbor in Deerfield, Illinois, which made a $3.6 billion bid that offered AHS stockholders $50 per share, compared with HCA's offer of $35. HCA reacted by threatening to drop its intravenous supply contracts with Baxter, worth about $100 million. Fences were mended when HCA agreed to step aside from the AHS merger for a cash payment of $150 million from Baxter (a breakup fee that Dr. Frist Jr. had negotiated as part of the AHS merger agreement just in case a company like Baxter were to show up later).[26] Putting that dollar amount in perspective, Vic Campbell said, "$150 million is almost as much as we made running hospitals [in 1985]. It came from a half a dozen of us working for six months, so it was a nice cash contribution for the company's hospitals."[27]

By early 1986 the company realized that the integration of hospitals and insurance wasn't a good long-term strategy. Campbell explained why hospital companies and HMOs didn't mix. "When a hospital company gets involved in the HMO business, it feeds customers through itself, but HMOs are profitable by limiting the amount of service. All of a sudden we were the HMO telling doctors that they needed to cut this and they needed to cut that. That is not something a hospital should be doing to its primary customer—the physician."[28]

Though Frist Jr. understood this disparity before HCA ventured into HMOs, the company pursued the insurance business at the time because, as Campbell said, "We thought maybe we were missing something. Wall Street was giving Humana this great stock multiple for being in the HMO business, so we decided to test it."[29]

The test didn't go well. "We came to the conclusion that we were not going to be an entire healthcare delivery and payment system within ourselves," said MacNaughton. "We decided that our primary role in the future would be to provide hospital care.... We were going to work with insurers for the most part rather than be insurers."[30]

In October 1986, HCA merged its insurance operations into Equicor, a new employee benefits company owned equally by HCA and The Equitable Life Assurance Society of the United States.[31] Ultimately, in March 1990, Equicor would be sold to Cigna for about $777 million.

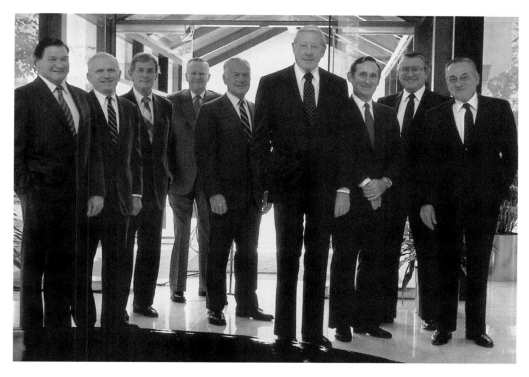

HCA's 1984 directors gather for group photos. Top (left to right): Carl E. Reichardt, chairman, president, and CEO of Wells Fargo & Company; Frank Borman, chairman, president, and CEO of Eastern Air Lines; Thomas N. P. Johns, M.D.; John D. deButts, retired chairman and CEO of AT&T; Owen B. Butler, chairman of Procter & Gamble; Donald S. MacNaughton, chairman of HCA; David G. Williamson Jr., executive vice president of HCA; Robert Anderson, chairman and CEO of Rockwell International; and Irving S. Shapiro, partner at Skadden, Arps, Slate, Meagher & Flom. Bottom left (left to right): Donald V. Seibert, retired chairman and CEO of J. C. Penney; Max M. Diamond, M.D.; Frank T. Cary, chairman of the executive committee of IBM; Charles J. Kane, chairman of Third National Corporation; Frank S. Royal, M.D.; and Joe B. Wyatt, chancellor of Vanderbilt University. Bottom right (left to right): Thomas F. Frist Jr., president and CEO of HCA; R. Clayton McWhorter, executive vice president of HCA; Barbara M. Clark, the Massey Companies; and Winfield Dunn, senior vice president of HCA.

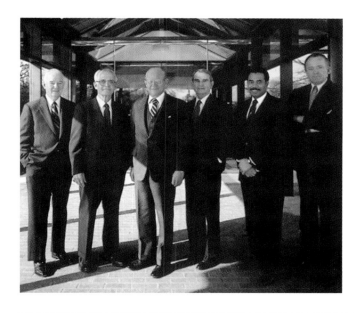

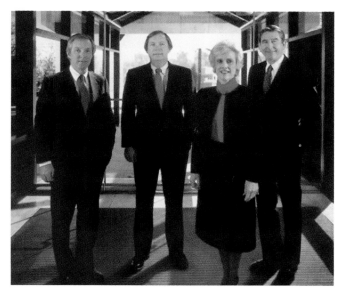

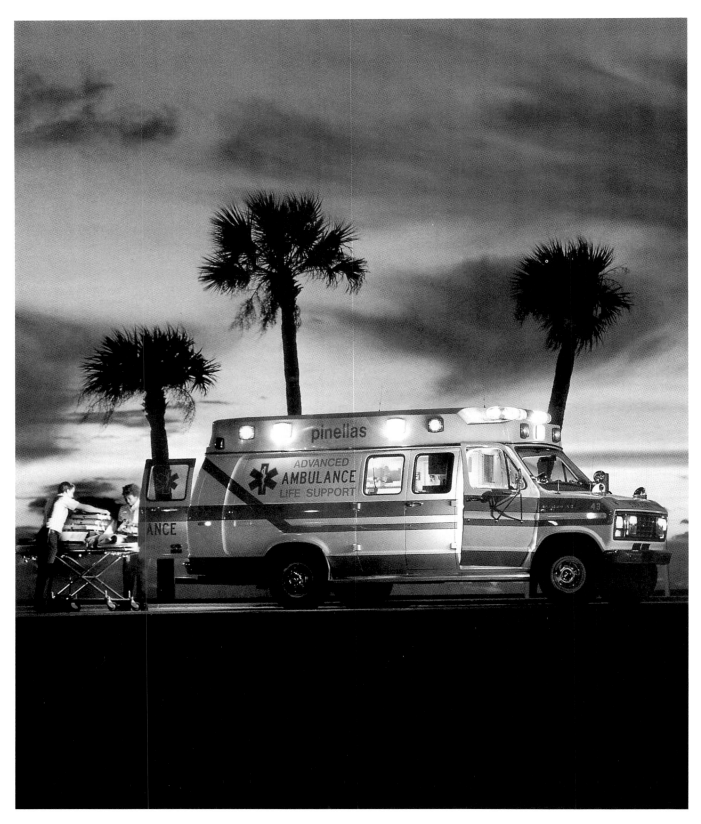

In 1976, HCA owned five medical transportation companies, which linked hospitals, physician offices, clinics, and other facilities with services ranging from nonemergency transfer to air ambulance life support.

CHAPTER FIVE

SHAKEOUT AND BUYOUT

1986–1989

*HCA's repositioning is a response to the tremendous changes which
began in the mid-1980s in the U.S. healthcare delivery system.*

—Thomas Frist Jr., 1987

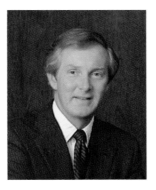

FOR THE FIRST TIME SINCE its founding 18 years earlier, HCA suffered an earnings decline in 1986 as the industry began transitioning from a cost-reimbursed industry. The transition began to take root in 1983, when the federal government made the most extensive revision of Medicare since the program began in 1965. Medicare reimbursements were now driven by diagnostic related groups (DRGs). Under the law's prospective payment system (PPS), hospitals could no longer charge Medicare according to their costs. Instead they would be reimbursed only a predetermined amount for a diagnosed illness. Initially, 467 DRGs were established. The DRG rates were to be adjusted upward each year based on the actual rate of hospital inflation.

Hospitals began phasing in the prospective payment system in October 1983, and at first the new system seemed to be working, both for HCA and for the federal healthcare budget. Indeed, management observed just that in the 1984 annual report, saying that HCA's earnings rose 20 percent while U.S. healthcare inflation for the past year had slowed to 6 percent, the lowest rate of increase since 1966.[1]

When DRGs were introduced, Vic Campbell noted that investors "loved it. . . . They saw it as a prospective reimbursement, not just a cost reimbursement. The law established incentives for those, like HCA, that were good at managing the cost side of the business."[2]

But the benefits of the new system didn't last. The prospective payment system had at first been a carrot, rewarding hospitals for greater efficiencies. But in the three years since its establishment, it became a stick, punishing them through costly, stringent regulations that were intended to cut healthcare costs.

In October 1985, the federal government froze Medicare payment rates to hospitals. From March through September of 1986, payments actually fell when Congress enacted the Gramm-Rudman-Hollings deficit-control measure. Ultimately, HCA suffered an 11 percent gap between the Medicare rates mandated in 1983 and their actual levels in 1986.

In the end, the federal government failed to live up to its promise to reimburse hospitals with reasonable payments for services rendered to Medicare beneficiaries. If a doctor ordered tests and procedures that caused the patient's bill to exceed Medicare's limit for a particular diagnosis, the physician, the hospital, private insurers—anybody other than Washington—had to pay that runover. HCA insisted that the policy jeopardized the quality of care in its hospitals.[3]

Dr. Frist Jr. led the HCA management team's 1989 leveraged buyout, which turned HCA into a privately owned company.

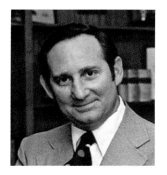

David G. Williamson Jr. became vice chairman of the board in 1985. He died a year later, on November 3, 1986. A room for visiting executives at HCA's corporate offices is named in his honor.

"Medicare reimbursement is extremely political," said Helen King Cummings, who as vice president of health financing was one of HCA's Medicare experts. "When you make changes to a global system like Medicare, you help a particular group of hospitals but hurt others. There are a lot of controversial issues. If Medicare pays for the extremely expensive cases, for example, then it's going to have less to pay for basic costs. If it pays doctors more, it pays hospitals less—because the pie is relatively fixed. You have to figure out how to divvy up the pieces."[4]

Not only did the government renege on its commitment to provide annual payment increases, but it also failed to eliminate the administrative burdens of cost reimbursement. "Everyone thought that after going on this prospective payment system, cost reports would go away," explained Trish Lindler, who joined HCA in 1975 and later became senior vice president for HCA's government programs. "Of course, they got even more complicated. The Mayo Foundation did a study and determined that there are 132,000 pages of Medicare regulations, which means they far surpass the tax code. That tells you the system is complicated."[5]

The new rules also intensified competition among hospitals for patients and capital and fed the demand for managed care programs. HMOs put pressure on hospitals to reduce costs, partially by restricting hospital admissions. More and more Americans were becoming enrolled in health maintenance organizations, and by the mid-1980s the rising number of HMOs began cutting into hospital occupancy rates.

HCA's "Black Monday"

It didn't take long for the Medicare freeze to wound HCA's earnings. HCA had scheduled a meeting with the investment community on the first Monday of October 1985 to give a routine update.

Over the weekend before, however, all of the hospitals had sent in their preliminary budgets for the coming year. The news was disturbing; it didn't appear likely that HCA's 1986 earnings could possibly live up to its historical 20+ percent growth.

"I was sitting with Tommy Frist and Sam Brooks, the chief financial officer, and we were trying to decide whether we really had enough information to make this determination," remembered Vic Campbell. "Should we wait awhile to get better information? Should we cancel the meeting with the investment community? On Sunday night, Tommy made the call that we would proceed. We'd tell people what we knew, that we foresaw we wouldn't make our earnings targets in 1986."[6]

When HCA acknowledged that it expected earnings to be flat in 1986—a shocking change from the company's typical annual growth of 20 to 25 percent—hospital stock prices tumbled. "Panic selling began," the *New York Times* reported, estimating that hospital chains collectively lost more than $1.5 billion in market value in one day. Todd B. Richter, an analyst with Morgan Stanley, said, "What happened can only be described as a bloodbath." And Margo Vignola at L. F. Rothschild, Unterberg, Towbin told the *Wall Street Journal*, "You're watching the biggest player in the industry stumble and crumble."[7]

It's worth noting that HCA took such a beating because it was the first public hospital company to recognize and tell investors that earnings would level out. Within a year's time, all other investor-owned hospital companies were forced to admit to lower-than-expected earnings. A few years later, investors voiced their appreciation to HCA for being the first to alert them. This was one of many times that HCA management was credited with telling the investment community and the general pubic about company and industry trends before they were widely known. After taking over as chairman and CEO in 2002, Jack Bovender was often quoted as saying, "Tell all you know, tell it as soon as you know it, and tell everyone who will listen."

Back to the Basics

HCA reemphasized its basic principles: quality care in both a clinical and a social sense and good relations with physicians and employees. "The things that made us good in the first place are going to continue to make us good in the future," said McWhorter in 1986, one year after he took HCA's presidential reins. "I'm an operations-oriented person. But I've picked up these philosophical thoughts [on the importance of quality and good relationships with doctors] through osmosis, by being around here with this team. And I think that my job now is to be sure that those philosophies are pushed on to others."[8]

HCA's reemphasis on its basic principles did not mean that the company had ever forsaken those principles. But with the growing number of HMOs, which most doctors resented because they put restrictions on the patient's healthcare, HCA wanted to assure doctors that it was willing to work with them, to be their partners, in order to deliver the best possible care. "Back to the basics means looking

at the social side of things," said McWhorter. "Relationships with physicians. Being kind. Telling our employees we love them. The personal side, the service side. All of our hospitals have clinical quality—good bricks and mortar and good technology and equipment. But what's going to make the difference? What sets HCA apart? People."[9]

In essence, HCA's original pro-physician philosophy fit the competitive environment. Dr. Frist Sr.'s serene presence fortified HCA's dedication to improving people's lives. "Like every-

Even through the turbulent 1980s, while HCA downsized and restructured through the LBO, the company retained its focus on providing physicians and hospital employees with the latest equipment and most up-to-date facilities.

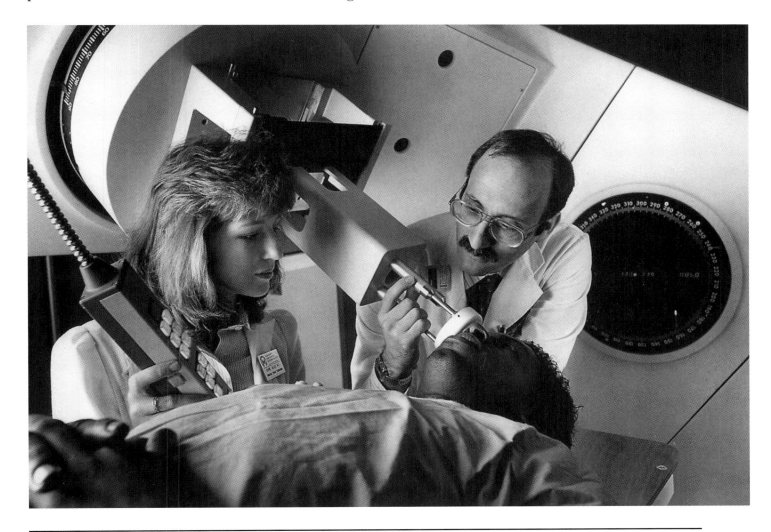

thing else in life, the healthcare field has peaks and valleys," he said in early 1987. "But what transcends all those peaks and valleys is the main thing our company was founded on—and that's the simple truths like character and family life, honesty and integrity, loyalty and persistence. The humanitarian philosophy of our company has taken us through hard times very successfully. And I think it will bring us out of the little valley in the healthcare field to a greater height than ever."[10]

The HealthTrust Spin-Off

At some point in 1986, it became clear to Frist Jr. that a dramatic restructuring or downsizing was necessary to reposition HCA, for internal operational improvements and in the eyes of investors. In the spring of 1987, HCA announced a plan to downsize from 230 hospitals to a core group of medical-surgical hospitals and psychiatric hospitals. Frist Jr.'s idea was to create a new Nashville-based company (subsequently named HealthTrust), which would acquire 104 hospitals from HCA for $1.7 billion in September 1987.[11]

HealthTrust was a new company principally owned by an employee stock ownership plan (ESOP) and headed by Clayton McWhorter as chairman and chief executive officer. Donald MacNaughton became chairman of HealthTrust's executive committee, and Charles N. Martin Jr., formerly HCA's executive vice president, became president and chief operating officer of HealthTrust.

As it did with future divestitures and spin-offs, HCA continued to provide systems and services to the sold facilities, recalled Tom Cato, HCA's chief information officer at the time.[12]

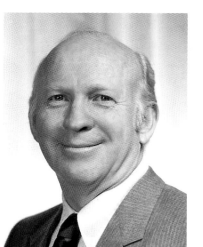

John Tobin, HCA's executive vice president of operations, was in charge of all hospital operations in 1985. Tobin joined HCA in 1971 as administrator of Johnston-Willis Hospital in Richmond, Virginia.

The facilities sold to HealthTrust were generally smaller and more rural than the larger, more urban hospitals retained by HCA. Together they accounted for only 20 percent of HCA's domestic revenues.[13] Jack Bovender, then HCA's president of group operations, said that, before HCA's restructuring, it had been "difficult to focus attention on individual hospitals because of our size. Now, resources and attention are more clearly focused. There's more flexibility and a feeling that individual hospitals will no longer get lost in a huge system."[14]

"We decided that maybe HCA was too big," McWhorter explained in 1987. "We'll have more leeway as a private company to do some things that the larger public system would not or could not do."[15]

HCA's decision to spin off the hospitals to a separate company benefited the people who worked in the hospitals as well as the hospitals themselves. Upon its creation, HealthTrust became the nation's largest employee-owned company. "When Congress studied employee stock ownership plans and passed legislation encouraging ESOPs, it was trying to foster programs like ours, in which the wealth of a company would be more equitably dispersed," said McWhorter.[16]

Though some analysts were skeptical of just how equitable HealthTrust would be for employees, HCA and HealthTrust executives were confident. "If our projections are correct," McWhorter told the *Washington Post,* "the return to the employee [through the ESOP] should be greater than what they would be getting presently."[17] Furthermore, many HCA employees who faced being laid off as a result of company budget cuts instead were able to retain their jobs under a new company's umbrella.

"By almost any yardstick, HealthTrust has performed better than most observers expected it could," wrote *Advantage* magazine in July 1990.[18]

HealthTrust stayed ahead of its debt repayment schedule, and by the first quarter of fiscal year 1990, it was able to report its first pretax profit, of $11.4 million.[19] In the words of HealthTrust president Charlie Martin, the company reached its financial goals by paying mind to "about a gazillion little individually insignificant things that in the aggregate got a good result."[20] This included good communication to employees about what an ESOP meant to them, which in turn resulted in employees giving their all to make the company a success. Though it was a private company, McWhorter said HealthTrust "acted like a public company from day one. . . . Openness has been an exceptionally good strategy for us."[21] In 1991 HealthTrust went public again, and by 1994 the company had reported net income of $122 million on revenues of $2.4 billion.[22]

Tender Offer

After the HealthTrust spin-off on September 17, 1987, HCA was nearly half the company it had been in number of hospitals, but it held a core group of 82 acute care and 50 psychiatric hospitals. HCA saw immediate improvement in its operational and financial strength.[23]

A key facet of HCA's restructuring involved a common stock repurchase program utilizing a significant portion of the cash proceeds it received from the HealthTrust sale. On the same day the HealthTrust spin-off was finalized, HCA invited shareholders to tender up to 12 million shares of common stock at prices from between $47 and $51 a share. (HCA stock was currently trading at $44.75.[24]) HCA intended to select a single purchase price within that range that would be sufficient to purchase the 12 million shares. The tender offer was to expire on October 19, but on October 14 the deadline was extended to allow shareholders an opportunity to review the company's favorable third-quarter results before making their decision. The new expiration date was set for October 22, 1987.[25]

When the stock market plummeted on "Black Monday," October 19, 1987, the company found its offer of $47 per share considerably above the new market price of about $30. HCA extended the expiration date again so it could assess how the stock market upheaval might affect its tender offer. On November 2, HCA determined that its finances and future prospects weren't impaired by the overall market decline and announced that it would live up to its legal and moral commitment to repurchase tendered shares at $47. "We're a company that honors

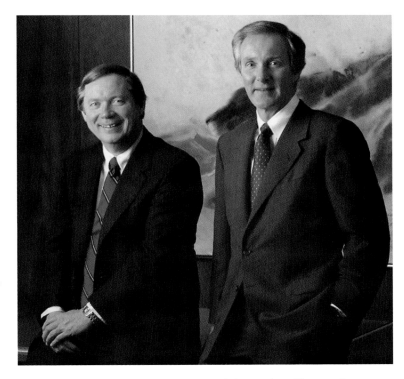

Clayton McWhorter (left), president and chief operating officer, and Thomas Frist Jr., chairman and chief executive officer, in 1986.

our commitments," said HCA Chief Financial Officer Roger E. Mick. "This allows shareholders to share in the $1.6 billion we received from the HealthTrust spin-off."[26]

HCA once again extended the expiration date, to January 4, 1988, to give shareholders adequate time to assess how the stock market crash affected their personal financial situations and to consider HCA's offer. On January 5, 1988, HCA completed the repurchase of 12 million shares for $564 million.[27]

The LBO

The late 1980s were a time of corporate takeovers and leveraged buyouts (LBOs). The junk bond market was at its height, with Michael Milken's Drexel Burnham leading the way. Takeover firms like Kohlberg Kravis Roberts & Company (KKR) and Forstman Little were cash rich and looking for undervalued (post–Black Monday) companies in all industries.

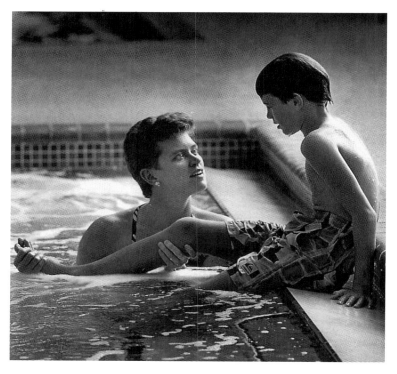

After the HealthTrust spin-off was complete, HCA's earnings were accelerating nicely, but its stock had moved up only slightly by the late summer of 1988, due primarily to the overall stock market weakness.[28] Years later, analyst John Hindelong called the hospital industry of the 1980s a "bloodletting." He remembered feeling frustrated by his inability to convince the investing public that HCA's stock was undervalued. "By the late 1980s, HCA's business had stabilized and had begun to show signs of improvement," he said. "But investors were still jaded by the [DRG freeze] of the mid-1980s."[29]

According to company documents, CFO Roger Mick, who served 22 years with HCA before retiring in 1992, first proposed a leveraged buyout

Above: Even after HCA downsized, it continued to meet two rapidly growing healthcare needs: rehabilitative services and psychiatric care.

Right: HCA's hospitals go beyond treating patients. They reach out to communities through wellness and preventive medicine programs such as this evening class in the Lamaze technique for natural childbirth.

(LBO) by management to Frist Jr. on August 1, 1988. It surprised few that HCA's chief executive was very receptive. Immediately, Mick, Frist Jr., and treasurer Bill McInnes began to put together the outside financial advisors needed to pull off a highly leveraged buyout. J. P. Morgan was retained as investment banker and financial advisor for Frist Jr.'s LBO team.

On Labor Day, Vic Campbell and Scott Mercy, who worked in HCA's investor relations department, checked into an obscure New York hotel and began working day and night with J. P. Morgan to prepare a memorandum outlining the terms of a management bid for the company.

Campbell recalled that no one other than Frist Jr., Mick, McInnes, and General Counsel Ron Soltman knew what he and Mercy were doing in New York. Many thought they were enjoying themselves at the U.S. Open Tennis Tournament in New York.[30]

On September 15, 1988, HCA announced that Frist Jr. and other senior executives were considering making an official offer to buy HCA for about $47 a share. HCA stock jumped from the low $30s, where it had been drifting, to almost $45.

It was a brave and risky venture. The buyers would need nearly $5 billion in financing by the time they bought HCA's equity and assumed more than $2 billion in existing debt.[31]

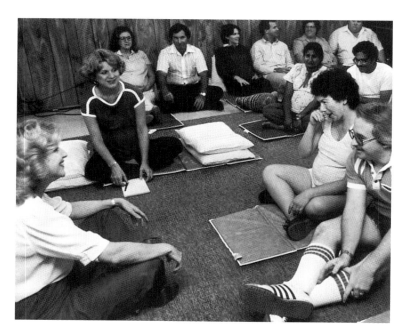

HCA's board formed an ad hoc special committee chaired by Irving Shapiro, which hired Morgan Stanley & Company as its financial advisor. On October 6, the special committee announced that if it received an official offer from management of $47, it would be rejected, but that the special committee was prepared to consider any proposal by management or others. A week later, the Frist group made a formal offer of $51 a share, to be financed by $43 in cash and $8 in unspecified securities.

On October 15, the special committee determined not to take action on management's offer, noting that it had received written indications from other parties that may have been prepared to offer more than $51 per share. The special committee extended the time period to submit offers to November 18.

Campbell, Mick, and Frist Jr. recalled that the wait from October 15 to November 18 was the longest 34 days of their lives. Campbell was assigned to coordinate due diligence sessions for other potential suitors. KKR was the most interested and the most focused. "One day I thought they would be a buyer—the next day I didn't," Campbell said. "My emotions went back and forth almost daily for a month."[32]

As for Frist Jr., he stood to lose the company that he and his father had spent 20 years building. Once HCA's board authorized the bid process, in effect, HCA was for sale to the highest bidder. Anyone with enough money could top management's offer—and many believed Humana, HCA's Louisville competitor, might try to trump Dr. Frist Jr.'s bid.[33]

Meanwhile, Wall Street and the financial world were fascinated by the fusillades flying fast in a different bidding war—the struggle for RJR Nabisco, the cigarette and cookie giant. In what became the largest LBO in American corporate history, KKR won the prize. KKR partner Henry Kravis and his staff had looked at HCA's books after the Frist group's offer but were mainly intent on their primary target and thus distracted. In the end, Humana also stayed out of the bidding.[34]

Frist Jr.'s team debated over that 34 days whether it should raise its $51 offer. In the end, Frist Jr. believed that $51 was the "right price"— a very good price for HCA shareholders and a

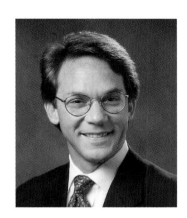

Scott Mercy, son of former senior vice president George Mercy, who died in 1980, joined HCA's investor relations department right out of college in 1983. He was a rising star at HCA, becoming one of the company's youngest senior officers in the mid-1990s. He chose to leave the company a few years after HCA merged with Columbia in 1993. In 1998 Frist Jr. asked Mercy to head HCA's rural hospital spin-off, LifePoint. Mercy died in a tragic private plane accident on May 30, 2000. He was 38.

price at which the buyers could afford to operate the company's hospitals without negatively impacting the quality of care being provided in local communities. Frist Jr.'s bid stayed at $51 and was presented in person to the full board in New York on Monday, November 21, 1988. No other bids came forth. Late that evening, the HCA board accepted the Frist group's offer, subject to shareholder approval.

Mick and Campbell recalled that it was an exciting ride from downtown Manhattan to the Teterboro, New Jersey, airport that night for Frist Jr. and his team—exciting, humbling, and somewhat frightening. They were about to borrow nearly $5 billion.[35]

To get the necessary loans, Dr. Frist Jr. pledged his entire net worth, and 21 officers who trusted their chief implicitly each put half of theirs on the line. The circle of new owners also included Goldman Sachs, J. P. Morgan, Rockefeller Capital, and Richard Rainwater. The new company would be 90 percent leveraged—$4.5 billion in debt—costing it $85,000 an hour in interest expense alone.[36]

In March 1989, Hospital Corporation of America became a private company. KKR's acquisition of RJR Nabisco, so fascinating to the press, closed within the same week. Frist Jr. happened to cross paths with KKR's Henry Kravis soon thereafter. Frist Jr. offered congratulations on RJR and asked why the Wall Street giant hadn't ultimately pursued HCA. "Tommy," Kravis replied, "I understand Oreo cookies a lot better than I do DRGs."[37]

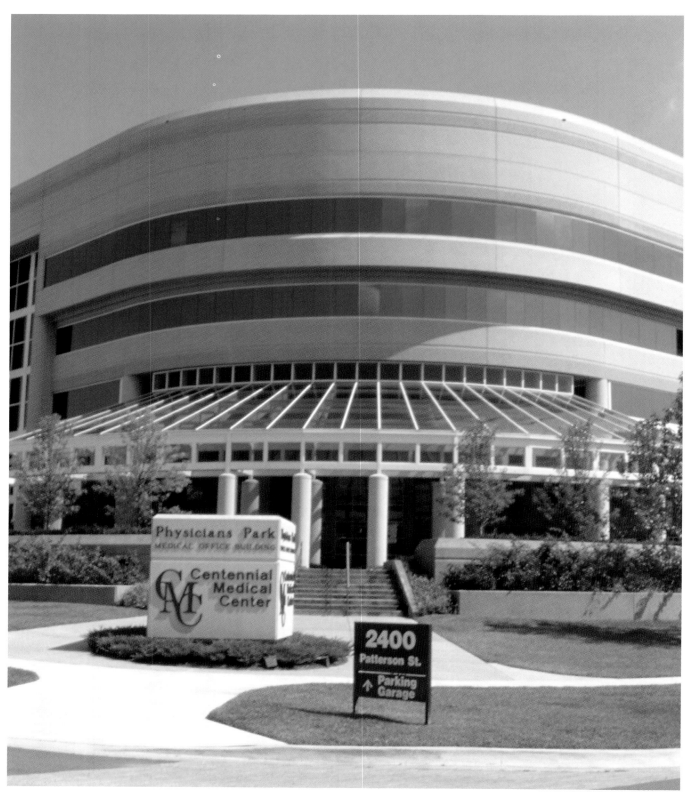

HCA's Centennial Medical Center in Nashville was formed when the old West Side, Park View, and Parthenon Pavilion hospitals were combined in 1990. The resulting 40-acre campus eventually had 685 beds, a physicians' park with 43 medical offices, and specialty services including The Sarah Cannon Cancer Center and the Women's Hospital at Centennial.

CHAPTER SIX

BACK TO THE BASICS

1989–1992

We didn't do the LBO out of greed or avarice. We did it to have control of our destiny.

—Thomas Frist Jr., 2001

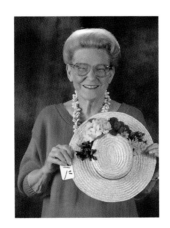

MANAGEMENT'S LEVERAGED buyout had been both "offensive and defensive," Frist Jr. once recalled, looking back on the heady days of the arbitragers and junk bond kings. "I knew we had to do some radical restructuring to the company, and it's easier to take those hits when you're a private company. It was defensive in that the public equity marketplace was not enamored with the hospital industry."[1]

Dr. Frist Jr. was convinced that Wall Street would change its tune about healthcare stocks generally and HCA in particular but that it might take three to five years for that to happen. In the meantime, the LBO group set about rebuilding HCA's core strength. The first and most pressing obligation was HCA's bridge loan—a $1.3 billion obligation that had to be repaid by March 1991. The strategy was to sell noncore assets to repay this debt.[2]

Paring Down

Around the world and close to home, "for sale" signs went up on HCA's noncore holdings and assets.

A clinical laboratory unit went for $44.6 million to a group of company executives who had managed it.

The hospital management subsidiary, holding 150 contracts, was sold to another such management group for $43 million and 10 percent stock interest and was renamed Quorum. Quorum was headed by longtime HCA executive Jim Dalton.

A partial sale of HCA's retained investment in HealthTrust brought $600 million in 1990. Two years later, HCA sold the rest of its investment in HealthTrust for $160 million. HealthTrust would later return to the HCA fold.

The Australian hospitals, laboratories, and clinical practices brought $83 million. These were the last of the company's overseas operations.[3]

The most valuable (at the time) noncore assets that HCA planned to sell—for $1.6 billion—were its psychiatric hospitals and drug treatment centers. The company had built the nation's largest chain of these, housing 6,000 beds. When HCA was ready to sell the assets in the spring of 1989, the psychiatric division had the highest operating margins of any division.[4]

HCA's Centennial Medical Center named its state-of-the-art cancer research and treatment center in Nashville after Sarah Cannon (pictured), known to millions of Grand Ole Opry fans worldwide as Minnie Pearl.

INFORMATION SERVICES

HCA REALIZED THE NEED TO CAPITAL-ize on the use of technology, and the company initially contracted with General Electric (GE) to custom design a system based on HCA's specific requirements. GE provided the data processing for each of the hospitals and allowed the company to easily consolidate information. GE provided computer services to HCA from 1973 to 1986.

As the company continued to grow, the computer industry was also undergoing a tremendous change. The computer companies had built excellent large mainframe computers and had started to build powerful mini and personal computers that could be connected. HCA recognized the value of this technology and invested in its own Information Services department. In 1985 HCA built a state-of-the-art Data Center that would provide the company with a valuable resource for years to come. HCA harnessed the power of the new, smaller computers and created software for each of the hospital departments. HCA linked the individual hospital systems together to improve operating efficiencies.

This technology decision allowed the company to build software that met the changing information requirements of each hospital. Also, HCA was a pioneer in electronically linking the physician offices to the hospitals. This consolidated all the information gathered at the individual hospitals by linking the hospital systems to the corporate mainframe computers and allowed information to be moved between computers.

HCA has had five chief information officers, or CIOs, during its history (Clovis Wood, Joe Hodge, Tom Cato, Rick Chapman, and Noel Williams), and each made significant contributions in using technology to meet HCA objectives.

Throughout its years as a private company, HCA continued to reinvest in facilities and equipment. It also continued to collect information from each of its regional healthcare systems for integration into its Data Center (atrium shown). The network system linked patient records with large data bases to improve hospital efficiency.

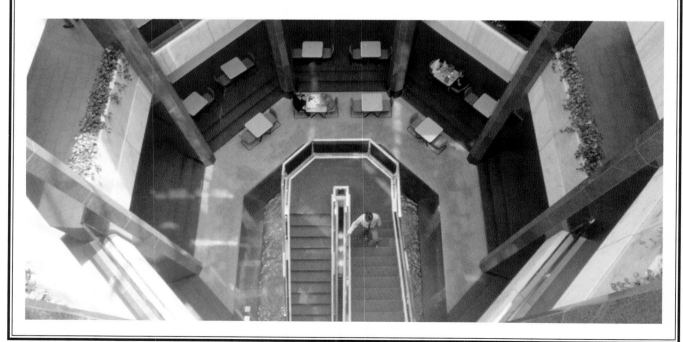

Dr. Frist Jr.'s idea was to sell HCA's psychiatric hospitals in the same way he had sold acute care facilities to HealthTrust back in 1987: to employees organized under a stock ownership plan (ESOP). HCA tried to interest major banks that might back a loan of more than $1 billion to the ESOP.[5]

An unfortunate burst of negative coverage in the nation's press about teenagers hospitalized for mental health set the plan back. Employers began to tighten up on behavioral and mental health benefits for their employees.[6] The financial press began to ask questions about HCA's planned transaction, beginning with an article in *Forbes* titled "A Crazy Deal?"

Despite the negative attention drawn to psychiatric care, by late September HCA had put together an equity and junk bond financing package with several large New York investment banking firms. However, in October the bottom dropped out of the junk bond market, and just before Christmas 1989 the plan fell through when lenders declined to fund the bid for the ESOP.[7]

Relief came unexpectedly. Cigna Corporation offered to buy HCA's 50 percent stake in its insurance subsidiary, Equicor, for $777 million cash. Suddenly the psychiatric deal was no longer critical to debt repayment. The company could adhere to its payment schedule with the proceeds from Cigna and the cash from a $545 million recapitalization.[8]

Road to Recovery

By the spring of 1990, the results of the leveraged buyout, divestitures, and cost-cutting looked promising. Operating income rose in double digits, and HCA even looked as if it might post a profit, something unheard of at debt-burdened LBOs for several years after the transaction.

While some wondered if debt service was forcing HCA to starve its spending for essentials, HCA was continuing to invest in facilities and equipment. Between 1989 and 1992, it invested $500 million on capital projects, with particular focus on expanding its hospitals' outpatient services. HCA's goal was to substantially increase—perhaps by as much as two-thirds—the revenue that outpatient facilities at HCA hospitals had generated before the buyout. By

1992 "same hospital" medical-surgical outpatient visits had increased 11 percent, generating net outpatient revenue growth of about 19 percent. Outpatient revenues represented nearly 30 percent of medical-surgical hospital net revenues.[9]

Debt service had consumed 15 cents of every revenue dollar when HCA first went private, but by the end of 1991 debt service was down to $.09 cents per revenue dollar. Additionally, HCA had cut operating costs enough to achieve annual savings of $70 million.[10] The owners could point to a solid record of achievements in their effort to put HCA on the road to recovery. Net operating revenues were climbing between 3 and 8 percent a year. Net operating revenues from inpatient services in particular increased 6 to 7 percent annually, and outpatient revenues climbed 19 to 20 percent. Interest expense decreased by $88 million in 1991 and $203 million in 1992. Debt as a percentage of total capital, which stood at 86 percent at the beginning of 1992, had fallen to 63 percent by year's end.[11]

"The leveraged buyout changed the whole complexion of the company," said Jack Bovender. "As a private company, we were off everybody's radar screen. We were just a great little company with wonderful hospitals."[12]

"The three years while we were a private company were very exciting," said Bill Rutherford, who joined the company in 1986 in the internal audit department and later became CFO for the company's Eastern Group. "We got really focused, and there was a lot of celebration, a lot of positive energy inside the organization. People really felt good about not only what we'd accomplished but where we were going."[13]

The LBO "was a great opportunity," added Richard Bracken, who at the time was CEO at HCA's Centennial Hospital (formerly Park View) in Nashville and later became HCA's president and chief operating officer. "It allowed us to rethink our operating priorities, and we became better operators and managers during that time."[14]

"The LBO is probably the most focused I have seen the company on executing an operating model," recalled Bruce Moore, who joined HCA in 1982 and later became senior vice president of operations administration. "Since we were not a publicly traded stock, one of our big challenges was effectively communicating to option holders and

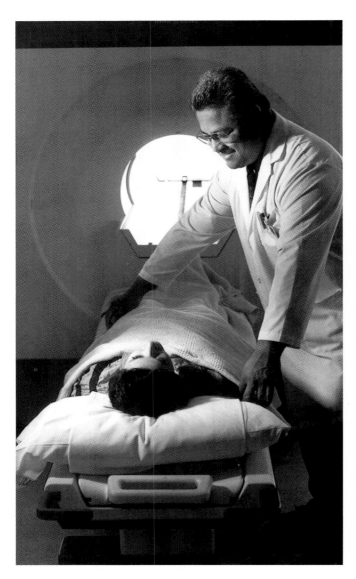

Both pages: HCA hospitals were equipped with the latest medical technologies, and having a soothing hospital atmosphere was of key importance, too. People wanted, as Jack Bovender, executive vice president and chief operating officer, pointed out, an "institution that makes their lives rewarding, pleasant, and satisfying."

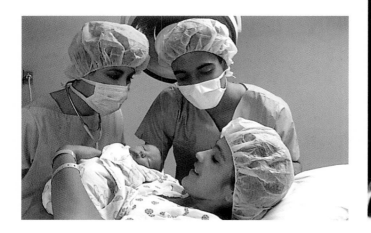

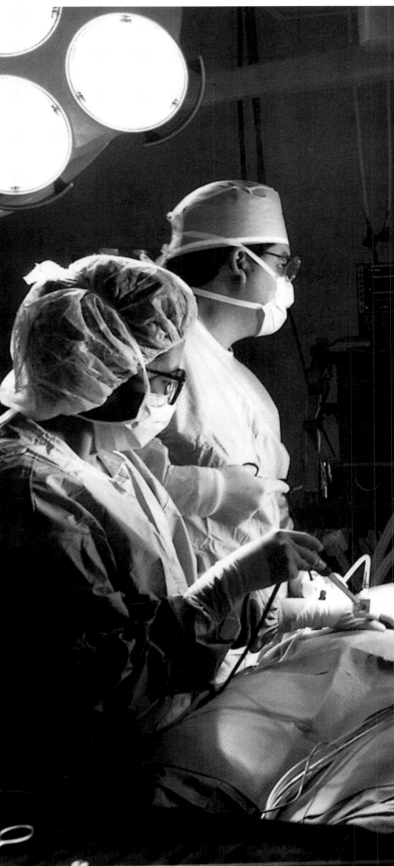

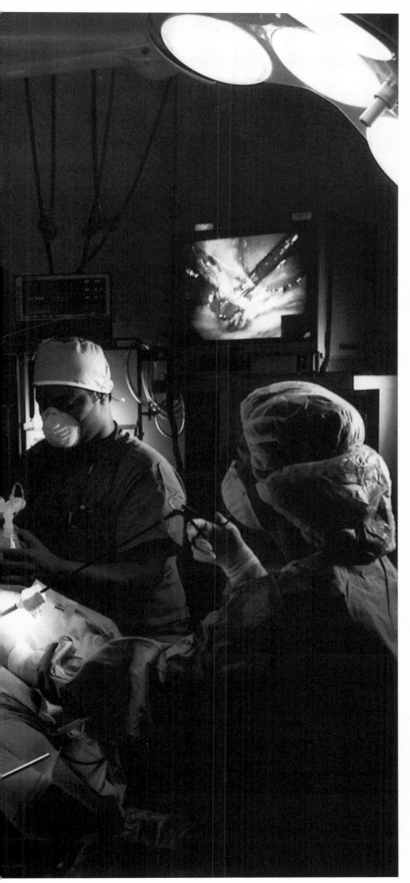

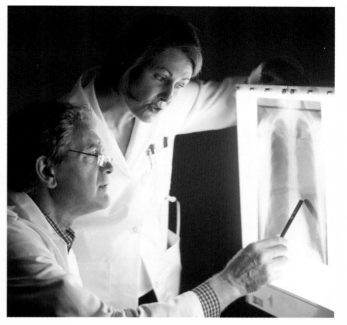

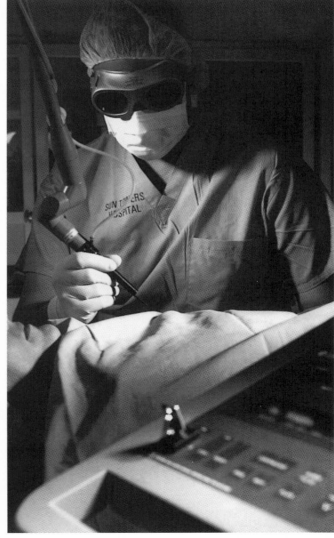

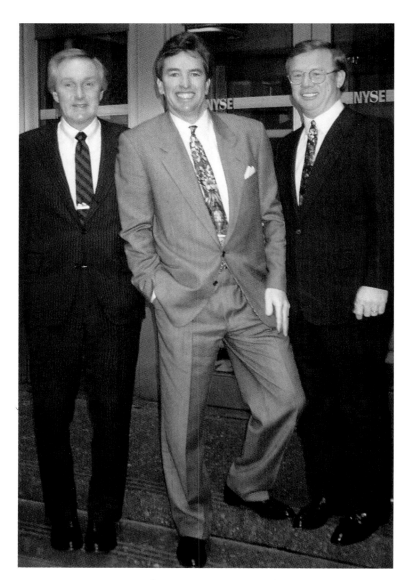

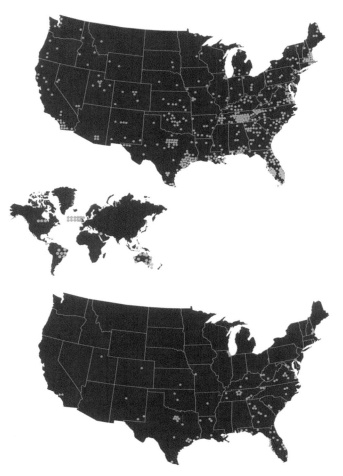

Left: Dr. Frist Jr., Vic Campbell, and Roger Mick had reason to smile. After a three-year LBO, the company returned to the New York Stock Exchange with an IPO in March 1992.

Below: In 1986, HCA owned or managed 486 hospitals around the world. By 1992, the year HCA that stock was once again traded publicly, the company owned 99 facilities, all in the United States.

retirement plan participants if value was truly being created from their efforts. Once we went public again, it became obvious."

Moore went on to discuss the lasting success of the LBO. "One of the best accounts of its success came from Graef Crystal, a nationally recognized compensation and executive accountability expert," Moore said. "When Crystal was testifying as a government expert at a General Accounting Office hearing in Washington, he said something to the effect that 'Dr. Frist Jr. had stepped up to the plate with his own money and knocked it out of the ballpark. In addition, every employee benefited since the retirement plan had been a major investor in the LBO. This is the American way.'"

Moreover, Moore said, "Tommy asked all 21 management investors, who benefited from the LBO's success, to establish a donor advisory fund through the Nashville Community Foundation, which continues to provide great benefits to the Nashville community."

For the buyout group—Dr. Frist Jr. and his management team, Goldman Sachs, J. P. Morgan, Rockefeller Capital, and Richard Rainwater—the three years of private ownership were golden. Their insiders' stake increased in value more than 700 percent, making their $283.7 million investment worth more than $2.3 billion. Stock options could be converted to shares worth hundreds of millions, and still the investment group would hold 75 percent control of HCA.[15]

Going Public—Again

On the first business day of 1992, HCA filed documents with the Securities and Exchange Commission to offer stock for public sale. The initial public offering (IPO) on March 4 would prove to be the second largest of the year, totaling approximately $700 million of common stock. The IPO comprised 34 million new shares, about one-fourth the total number of shares in the company. The opening price was $21.50.[16]

HCA saw considerable benefits in a return to the public market, including a lower cost of capital, greater financial flexibility, more dollars available for investment, and liquidity for nonmanagement investors J. P. Morgan, Goldman Sachs, Richard Rainwater, and others. It emphasized that these dollars would be spent to "further develop the growth of our existing hospitals."[17]

Lower interest rates and the once-again-bullish attitude toward healthcare stocks led most to predict a rosy future for the new publicly traded HCA. One reporter put it this way:

> *For sale: stock in cyclical business with a leveraged buyout in its past. Knocked around by recession and debt. Eager to mend its ways. Could make big profits if economy revives.*[18]

For HCA's part, managers were convinced that they "had the right hospitals in the right markets with the right local strategies." In 1986, the year retrenchment began, the company owned or managed more than 480 healthcare facilities around the world. By the end of 1992, it owned 73 medical-surgical and 26 psychiatric hospitals. All facilities were in the United States; none was managed for another owner. "Focus" and "cash" were now the watchwords that "growth" had once been. The company believed that its future success depended upon being able to "demonstrate clinically successful patient outcomes at competitive prices."[19]

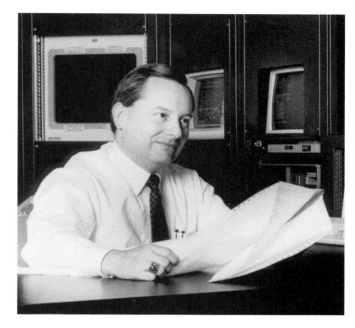

Jack Bovender, shown here as president of group operations in 1987, became executive vice president and chief operating officer in 1992. Later, he succeeded Frist Jr. as chairman and CEO.

In the fall of 1992, HCA's board tapped Jack O. Bovender Jr. to be executive vice president and chief operating officer. Bovender had been senior vice president and president of Eastern Group operations.[20]

An astute observer of changes afoot in American healthcare, Bovender also saw important continuities. "I am convinced that the hospital in each community holds the key to its own survival, as it always has," he had told an academic audience in 1986. There was no substitute for the well-run, efficient hospital oriented to consumers, he said. And who was the most important consumer? The doctor, of course.

He continued: "The overwhelming majority of our patients are directed to our institutions by physicians.... They will choose the institution that creates an atmosphere . . . that makes their lives rewarding, pleasant, and satisfying."[21]

It was a view that harkened back to the company's earliest days: make HCA hospitals places where doctors want to practice and to refer patients, and all else will follow.

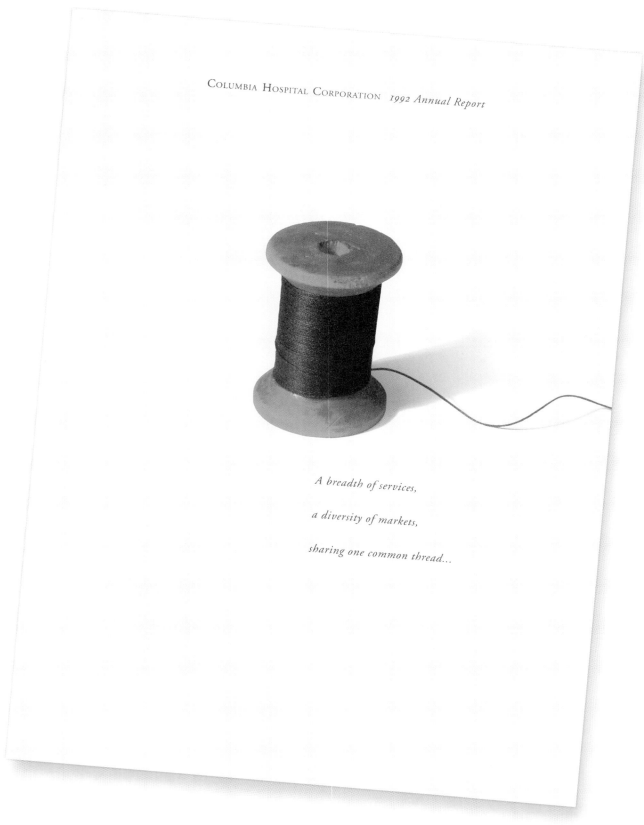

COLUMBIA HOSPITAL CORPORATION *1992 Annual Report*

A breadth of services,

a diversity of markets,

sharing one common thread...

Columbia Hospital Corporation, founded in 1987, grabbed national headlines in 1993 when it purchased Galen Health Care, a spin-off of Humana that was nearly four times the size of Columbia.

CHAPTER SEVEN

GREAT ASSETS MERGE

1993–1994

*We saw in Scott a new person who would be able to consolidate
all those assets—HCA, Galen, and Columbia, to start.*

—Thomas Frist Jr., 1994

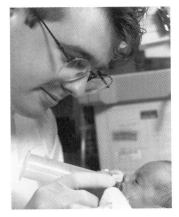

I N SELLING HCA'S NONCORE facilities, paring down its debt, and taking it public, Dr. Frist Jr. preserved his company's preeminent position in the investor-owned hospital industry. Burdened with $5.7 billion in debt at the time of the leveraged buyout—$90 of debt for every $10 of assets—Frist Jr. had pulled off a miraculous turnaround, not to mention one of the most successful management-led LBOs in the history of corporate America.

Unfortunately, as the nation's healthcare system moved more and more toward managed care and fixed reimbursements, investor-owned hospital companies like HCA had to look for ways to lower prices while still providing quality care and earning reasonable profits.

Columbia on the Map

Meanwhile, Humana had come to the same conclusion that HCA had reached a few years before: mixing insurance and hospitals was not working. David Jones, chairman of Humana, approached Dr. Frist Jr. in 1992 about buying Humana's hospitals, but the HCA executive decided the time was not right. It was difficult for Frist Jr. to turn down Jones's offer (Frist Jr. had always respected Humana's hospitals, and most industry observers rated Humana's hospital group

second only to HCA's), but having just become a public company again, HCA had made a commitment to its shareholders that it would deleverage over the next few years by paying down debt. Jones subsequently split his company into an insurance company, which retained the name Humana, and a hospital company, which adopted the name Galen from a physician of ancient Greece often regarded as one of the founders of medicine.[1] But this split was to be only an interim step in Humana and Galen's metamorphosis.

In September 1993, Texas-based Columbia Hospital Corporation, founded in 1987 by Rick Scott and Richard Rainwater, acquired Galen Health Care and moved Columbia's Fort Worth, Texas, headquarters to Louisville, Kentucky, where Galen was based. At the time of the purchase, Galen consisted of 74 hospitals and had $4 billion in revenues.[2]

"The deal with Columbia was conceived and implemented pretty quickly," said David Anderson, who was CFO of Galen when Columbia acquired it and would later become senior vice president

Therapists need extensive advanced training and dedication to teach a newborn in intensive care to feed.

COLUMBIA'S BEGINNINGS

COLUMBIA HOSPITAL CORPORATION was founded in October 1987 by Richard L. Scott, a young healthcare transaction lawyer in Dallas's largest law firm, and Richard Rainwater, a Texas investor who in 1989 became an HCA board member. (Rainwater told Frist Jr. at the time of the HCA LBO in 1989 that he was involved in a small start-up healthcare company.) In 1987 Scott had been one of three who indicated an interest in buying HCA, but HCA's board had rebuffed the offer, finding it not credible.

Scott recognized that the two largest hospital companies were not interested in acquisitions; in fact, they were net sellers of hospitals. So he figured that now was a great time to start a new company founded solely on acquiring hospitals. He began writing letters to owners of hospitals he thought might be open to a sale, mailing out a thousand inquiries in November alone. Ironically, his first purchase was in El Paso, where he (along with doctor-partners) bought two hospitals from HealthTrust, the company that HCA had spun off in the spring of 1987.[1]

Columbia's strategy was to quickly acquire hospitals and other healthcare services, link the various pieces together to make it easier for HMOs or employers to purchase all their healthcare needs from one source, and brand the company so that people would think of Columbia as the best place to go for healthcare services. Columbia wanted to offer everything to every prospective patient or client in each market. Scott also wanted to syndicate hospital ownership to local physicians.[2]

By 1990, Columbia served four markets—El Paso, Corpus Christi, Houston, and South Florida—and had grown to 13 hospitals and $290 million in revenues. It soon enjoyed the highest market share of any provider in El Paso and became a large provider of acute care services in Miami.[3] In May 1990, Columbia went public through the merger with publicly traded Smith Laboratories.[4] In the summer of 1992, Columbia bought Basic American Medical (BAMI), a small chain of eight hospitals with headquarters in Indianapolis.

After the purchase of BAMI, *Fortune* named Columbia the 12th-fastest-growing company in the nation. Columbia was thus slipping its regional identity and becoming a national chain.[5] But it was the Galen acquisition in September 1993 that put Columbia in the big leagues.

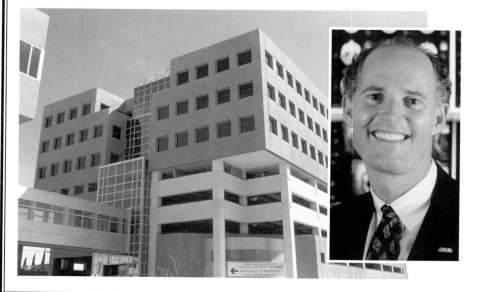

Inset: Chairman and CEO of Columbia Hospital Corporation Richard L. Scott

Left: Sun Towers Hospital and Sun Towers Behavioral Health Center in El Paso, Texas, were among the 94 hospitals Columbia brought into the merger with HCA. Most of Columbia's holdings before the merger were in Texas and Florida. Sun Towers Hospital, an acute care facility, had the only burn unit and lithotripter in the El Paso area.

and treasurer of HCA. "Columbia was a small company with a very high cost of capital, and Galen was a large company with an investment-grade balance sheet. We were an A-rated credit with a solid balance sheet and good cash flow, but we frankly struggled a bit in terms of what our operating strategy was going to be [after splitting from Humana]. A merger was a viable alternative for Galen, and Columbia seemed like a logical buyer. It seemed to be synergistic for both sides," Anderson recalled.[3]

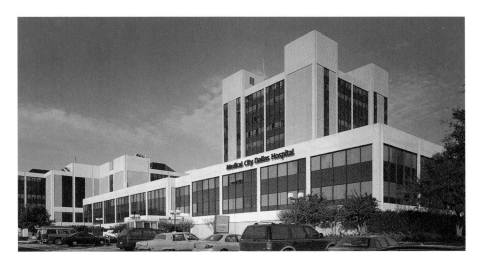

Medical City Dallas Hospital, one of the many facilities that came to Columbia via the Galen merger, remains one of the Dallas–Fort Worth area's premier hospitals.

Galen, four times the size of Columbia, brought Columbia's reach to almost a dozen new cities: Anchorage, Chicago, Dallas, Denver, Las Vegas, Los Angeles, Louisville, Montgomery, Orlando, Phoenix, and San Antonio. In several cities, including Corpus Christi, Houston, and Miami, both companies operated hospitals.

"All of a sudden, Columbia morphed into a very large organization that had a tremendous capacity to borrow money," said Anderson.[4] Indeed, the ink was barely dry on the final documents with Galen when Scott vowed to acquire 100 hospitals a year all around the country for the next five years.[5]

Rosalyn "Ros" Elton, who began working in El Paso in 1988 and later became a Columbia vice president and an HCA senior vice president, described the culture shock of Columbia's rapid growth. "I don't think anybody thought we were going to spring from the 23 hospitals we had in 1993 to having a hundred and some hospitals when we finished the merger with Galen," she said. "It was a totally different world. We didn't have a small company anymore."[6]

Scott now had the full attention of analysts on Wall Street. Consolidation was something they liked, and the necessity to cut costs was driving consolidation throughout healthcare. Doctors were forming or being pushed into alliances. Hospitals were sharing services and collaborating informally in new ways.[7]

As numbers of hospitals, admissions, and beds in service continued to fall nationwide, hospital boards increasingly felt the need to consolidate. The only question was whether their hospital would be the consolidator or the "consolidatee." Rick Scott was determined to be the consolidator. In city after city, his acquisition and regional managers pressed forward, contacting doctors, trustees, and administrators and offering to buy all or part of their facilities. David Vandewater, who worked at Scott's side as chief operating officer from 1991 until 1997, put the matter simply: In looking for prospects in Florida, "we put down a list of hospitals we wanted to buy. We got them."[8]

Some saw Scott as flash, but even Scott's detractors acknowledged his enormous energy, drive, and tenacity. He was seen as a visionary with free-market answers for the American healthcare system in the throes of painful change. Scott's unrelenting drive and work ethic took him to the summit of the investor-owned hospital industry.

Cause and Effect

Dr. Frist Jr. had been sorely disappointed that HCA had not been in a position to acquire Galen, for he considered the former Humana hospitals a great fit with HCA's hospitals in terms of their quality and location. Also, First Lady Hillary Clinton's proposed healthcare reform plan had begun to cast a cloud over the industry, and HCA's stock was stagnant. HCA needed to grow in order to compete in the new healthcare environment, but it was trading at only 11 times its earnings, and its PE ratio wasn't high enough to acquire other hospital companies. Columbia, having just acquired Galen, was trading at about 20 times its earnings. Frist Jr. saw a merger with Columbia as a good way to add prime assets while increasing its PE multiple. Also, the combined market cap of Columbia and HCA would provide instantaneous liquidity at a premium for HCA's largest shareholder, J. P. Morgan.

With the Clinton healthcare reform proposal looming, the idea made even more sense.

The plan set out to inject the federal government, and its controls, into each and every facet of healthcare, in effect usurping the role insurance companies had acquired over the years in controlling medical costs and availability. For starters, the sweeping revisions would mandate how physicians and hospitals were paid, imposing limits and perhaps forcing doctors to become involved in HMOs. Health plans would be required to meet federal standards for solvency. Physicians and hospitals would not be permitted to bill individuals for unpaid claims. Plans whose proposed premiums exceeded allowed rates would be required to accept lower premiums, and health plan providers would have to adjust payment rates or accept lower profits to make up the difference. Physician-hospital organizations (PHOs) teamed large numbers of hospitals with local doctors who would bargain with insurance companies to provide "womb-to-tomb" care. These PHOs were seen as potential winners under the new system.

On September 1, 1993, the day that Columbia acquired Galen, Dr. Frist Jr. called Richard Rainwater and suggested that it might make sense to merge Columbia and HCA. The next day, Rainwater brought Rick Scott into the conversation. Throughout September, the leaders hammered out the details, with Frist Jr. working to get the best price for HCA shareholders. He was successful. When the deal was struck on October 2, 1993, the negotiated price was 40 percent higher than HCA's current stock price. Scott would become president and CEO of the new entity, and Frist Jr. would be nonexecutive chairman.

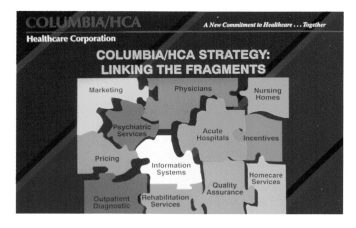

In the 1993 annual report, the newly formed Columbia/HCA Healthcare Corporation explained its strategy for linking components of the healthcare marketplace to make it "easier for larger purchasers of healthcare services to purchase all their healthcare needs from one source."

"[Scott] has the vision. He has the strategy. He's implementing it as well as anyone," Frist Jr. told the press.[9] He also pointed out that, in selling his business, he was following the blueprint of the Clinton plan (a draft of which he had seen just weeks before) to form alliances of providers who in turn would set up networks that attracted purchasers of healthcare. He also saw in Scott "a new person who would be able to consolidate all those assets—HCA, Galen, and Columbia, to start."[10]

Mega Merger

Columbia operated 94 general and specialty hospitals with 21,627 beds. HCA operated 96 general and specialty hospitals, with 20,485 beds. Both companies also operated diagnostic, outpatient, and other treatment centers. The new Columbia/HCA Healthcare Corporation with 190 facilities and more than 42,000 beds, became the largest investor-owned hospital firm in the world, employing 125,000 people in 26 states.[11]

The value of the Columbia/HCA deal was $10.25 billion, making it the seventh-largest merger in American industry since 1981. The new company would be in a position to effect major cost reductions. Scott estimated Columbia/HCA would save $138 million a year by combining marketing, data processing, and purchasing and by achieving more favorable lending rates on borrowed money. All would be accomplished by a tax-free exchange of shares, with no cash involved.[12]

Columbia's future looked bright. The new company, with entrepreneurial energy and free-market enterprise, was poised to capture opportunities in the roiling healthcare field. With the inking of the deal, it would have leading hospital positions in Houston, Miami, and many other major markets.[13]

Columbia seemed to have anticipated the key elements of the Clinton administration healthcare plan and was already stepping out front, achieving the plan's goals through market forces, not regulation. The administration favored networking and consolidation, and Rick Scott had accomplished these *en fine:* buy acute care hospitals and make them the base of operations in a local market. From there, acquire psychiatric hospitals, home healthcare companies, outpatient surgery clinics, and any other operation that the local manager believed would give Columbia the full continuum of care in the market. The company would offer one-stop shopping for managed care operators and, eventually, for the regional health alliances that the "National Health Security Act" proposed. "Move over, Hillary," one observer wrote, "Rick Scott is about to reform American healthcare."[14]

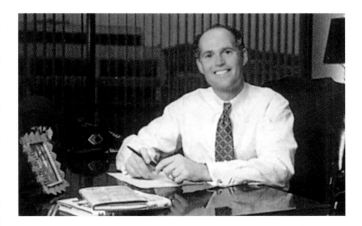

On February 10, 1994, the merger of Columbia Hospital Corporation and Hospital Corporation of America was finalized, and the world's largest healthcare provider was formed. Richard L. Scott, the president and CEO, would lead the company from his office in Nashville, Tennessee.

The challenge to Columbia was how to offer the smorgasbord of services in every local market that would win contracts from managed care outfits. "Giant hospital chain." "Tough tactics." "Fast growth." All those terms became associated with Columbia as early as the summer of 1994.[15]

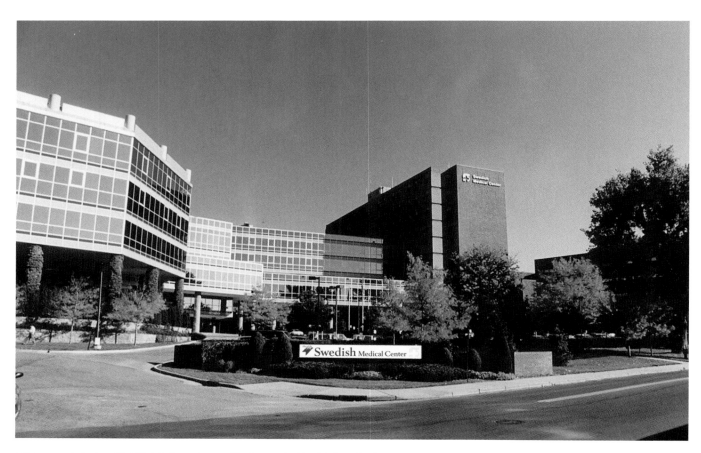

HCA completed a 50-50 joint venture with Denver's HealthOne in October 1995. The venture brought together six HealthOne hospitals, including Swedish Medical Center (pictured), and four HCA hospitals to create Colorado's premier hospital system.

CHAPTER EIGHT

SIZE AND BRANDING CREATE A LIGHTNING ROD

1994–1996

We will market health services under the Columbia brand. We will eagerly strive to build a household name to be synonymous with quality patient care, both nationally and locally.

—Richard L. Scott, 1995

RICK SCOTT CHARGED Columbia with energy and excitement. Under his leadership, the company experienced amazing growth. It went from operating 320 hospitals and approximately 125 outpatient centers in 1994 to operating 343 hospitals, 136 outpatient centers, and approximately 550 home health locations in 1996.

After merging with Galen and HCA, Columbia bought Medical Care America (MCA) for $850 million in September 1994. MCA was the nation's largest outpatient surgery chain, operating about 100 such centers, most of them in Columbia's existing markets. Integrating the surgery centers into its existing network significantly expanded Columbia's scope of services and helped it lower costs for outpatient surgical procedures.[1]

Later that year, Columbia moved to acquire HCA's spin-off company, HealthTrust. Others were bidding for the Nashville-based chain, which operated 119 hospitals, most of them in rural locations. But Rick Scott and Frist Jr. upped their offer against the competitors and successfully struck the deal for $5.6 billion, the largest merger in the history of investor-owned hospital companies. McWhorter became chairman of Columbia when the merger was completed in April 1995 (with Frist Jr. as vice chairman) but retired in May 1996 after a year of transition.[2]

At the time of the merger between HCA and Columbia, Rick Scott and Richard Rainwater had privately committed to moving the Columbia/HCA headquarters from Louisville to Nashville. A key result of the HealthTrust deal was the acceleration of these plans. Nashville had been the base of HCA's and HealthTrust's operations; the infrastructure was there (including the HCA Data Center). Tommy Frist Jr. thought that if the Columbia/HCA merger were to be successful over the long term, the headquarters should be in Nashville, where the infrastructure was and where a more stable corporate culture was in place.

The rapid succession of mergers during this period brought many of the hospitals from HCA's origins back to the company. These hospitals would later form the core of HCA's operations. "These hospitals represent the finest group of healthcare assets ever assembled in one company," Dr. Frist Jr. would later note.

Deals with Not-for-Profits

Combining the focus and energy of Rick Scott with the many years of industry credibility of the Drs. Frist and HCA positioned Columbia/HCA as a desirable acquirer or partner for many highly respected not-for-profit hospitals. In 1995 alone, Columbia acquired or formed joint ventures with 32 nonprofit hospitals.[3]

By forming a joint venture with Columbia, for example, Southwest Texas Methodist Hospital—

the largest, most widely respected, and most successful facility in greater San Antonio—was able to save more than $5 million in a single year through Columbia's purchasing power and new information systems.[4]

Likewise, Tulane University Hospital and Clinic, in New Orleans, was facing new market pressures and decided to join Columbia's network in order to reduce costs and expand opportunities for tertiary care referrals. Tulane was expected to save up to $5 million a year from Columbia's group purchasing contracts and consolidation of services with other Columbia facilities in New Orleans.[5]

Columbia acquired or formed joint ventures with other nonprofit hospitals, including Grant Hospital in Chicago; Independence Regional Medical

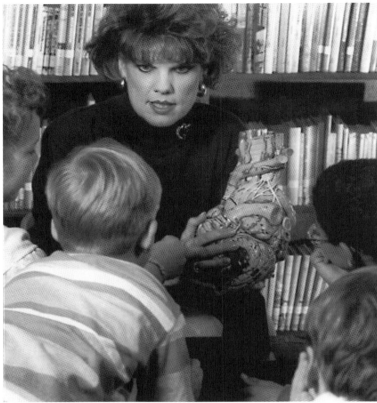

Center in Kansas City; MetroWest Medical Center in Boston; Winter Park Memorial Hospital in Orlando; Saint Joseph's Hospital in Fort Worth; Rapides Regional Medical Center in Alexandria; Memorial Healthcare System in Jacksonville; HealthOne in Denver; and Sisters of Charity of Saint Augustine, which had hospitals in Cleveland, Ohio, and Columbia, South Carolina.[6]

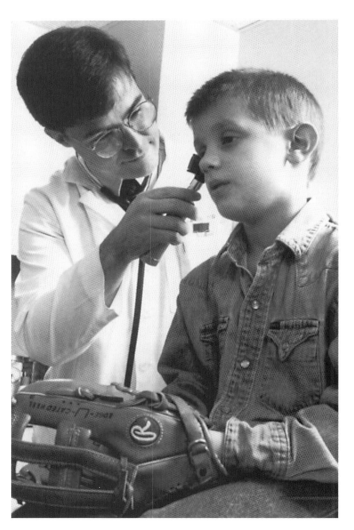

Above: In 1994 Columbia formed a joint venture with Rapides Regional Medical Center. The Rapides Foundation donated $1 million to the residency program of Louisiana State University's Medical School to educate family practitioners in central Louisiana.

Left: Rapides was committed to extending hospital educational programs to members of the community.

Opposite: In 1994 Columbia started operating Tulane University Hospital and Clinic in New Orleans. Tulane Hospital for Children, an affiliate of Tulane University Hospital, is a stand-alone specialty facility.

Praise and Criticism

While it made economic sense and was a natural offshoot of the changes coming to healthcare, Columbia's acquisition of not-for-profit hospitals sometimes met with suspicion. Local hospitals were seen by many as part of the local culture, hometown institutions where family members, friends, and neighbors were born, cared for, and died.

Since its beginnings 30 years before, the investor-owned hospital business had had its critics in Washington, both in the halls of Congress and in the bureaucratic warrens along Pennsylvania Avenue. In the past decade, they had gained credibility and respect, but Columbia's sheer size lit up Washington's radar screen; it was under constant, relentless scrutiny. The Federal Trade Commission closely examined its mergers, occasionally blocking an acquisition or ordering the company to divest itself of a certain number of holdings when it expanded into a new area. And while federal guidelines permitted doctors to acquire interests in a Columbia regional network, some members of Congress cast baleful glances at such arrangements and drafted legislation to curtail or abolish them.[7]

The press's scrutiny of Columbia was particularly intense as the company began seeking to acquire hospitals in communities and states where investor-owned hospitals had not previously operated. While 15 percent of hospitals were investor-owned, the hospitals were primarily in the South and West. Columbia met with increasing resistance as it entered northeastern and midwestern cities like Boston, Cleveland, and Chicago.

Still, investor-owned hospitals provided a dose of the right medicine for some markets. Aside from bringing capital and efficiencies to otherwise struggling hospitals, Columbia's entry into a locale provided great benefits to local communities through property and income taxes. Its arrival almost always led other providers to create new alliances. For example, when Columbia bought four hospitals in Orlando, Florida, in 1994, the city's two not-for-profit facilities rushed to integrate clinical services. Doctors also took notice. A group of 27 primary care physicians set up a "clinic without walls," a sort of merger that allowed them to use a common general ledger. Separately, a set of cardiologists formed a network to secure HMO contracts.[8]

Wall Street analysts gave Columbia high marks for eliminating duplicate operations and closing beds and, sometimes, facilities. It was the natural and necessary outcome of the managed care revolution, and it proceeded apace while Congress

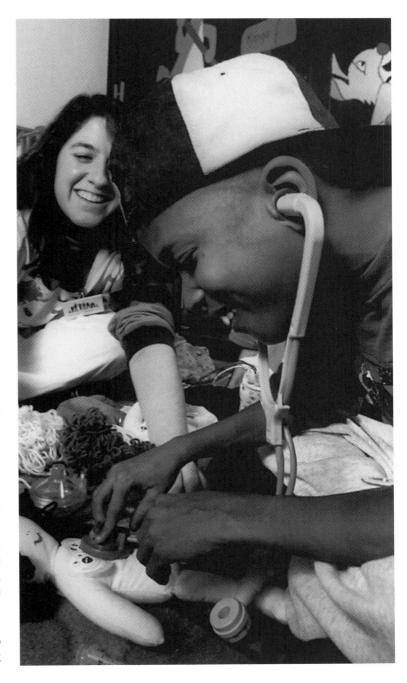

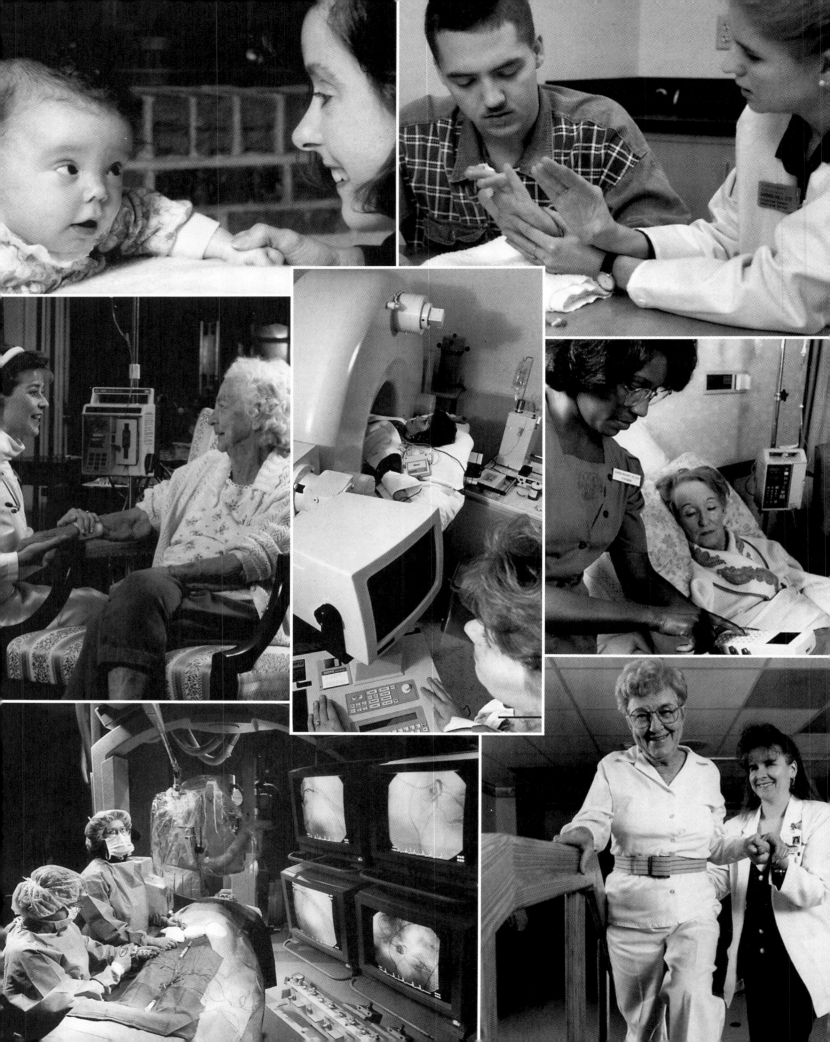

and President Clinton shadowboxed over how to deliver universal healthcare while reducing Medicare outlays.[9]

Becoming Too Big

In the winter of 1995–96, Columbia stood on the heights. It was the nation's ninth-largest employer, with some 285,000 people on the payroll, more than at General Electric or McDonald's.[10] In 1995 a study published by HCIA and Mercer Healthcare listed 30 Columbia hospitals among the nation's top 100 hospitals. Gallup polls found that Columbia hospitals had a 94 percent patient satisfaction rate, with the industry average being 88 percent. And 43 percent of Columbia hospitals surveyed by the Joint Commission for the Accreditation of Healthcare Organizations received "accreditation with commendation," when only 12 percent of all hospitals surveyed in 1995 received such recognition.[11]

With 326 hospitals and more than 100 outpatient surgery centers, as well as home health services, Columbia was also the nation's largest provider of healthcare services. Its admissions were increasing, as was its net income and the value of its shares. It anticipated adding 18 hospitals in 1996, had letters of intent with a score of other facilities, and was in discussions with many more. To be sure, Columbia owned only about 3 percent of total U.S. hospital facilities and was concentrated mainly in the South and Southwest, but it was exercising an influence out of proportion with these numbers.[12]

Rick Scott was admired by many for his vision of the future of American healthcare. He was called by some "the Bill Gates of healthcare."[13]

While Columbia's growth was lauded by many, some who had always harbored doubts or were threatened by investor-owned hospitals began to raise public concern that Columbia was getting too big. Consumer criticism escalated, legal challenges multiplied, and federal and state bureaucrats turned a baleful eye on Columbia.

Opposite: Columbia offered a comprehensive network of cost-effective, quality medical services.

In the late summer of 1996, a state court judge in Lansing, Michigan, ruled that under the state's laws, assets from charitable, nonprofit institutions could not be mingled with those of for-profit concerns like Columbia, which was pursuing an acquisition in Michigan. "The court's decision protects the fruits of charity from greed," Michigan's attorney general said. Church and consumer groups also hailed the ruling.[14]

On the West Coast, Columbia sought to buy four hospitals and the medical groups associated with San Diego's not-for-profit Sharp HealthCare. Attorney General Dan Lungren, later a candidate for governor, declared that Sharp's directors had greatly undervalued its holdings, based on higher prices offered by Columbia competitors. Sharp responded with specific concerns that had led it to reject the bids from those companies. Lungren nonetheless warned that he would "seek to hold the Sharp directors who voted to approve this transaction personally liable" for the difference.[15]

His stern words, picked up by national press, imperiled other deals in California and beyond, where attorneys general, regulators, and hometown advocates for local hospitals were stirring. Columbia's competitiveness, aggressive self-promotion, and numerous acquisitions generated deep emotions, state senator Diane Watson (Democrat-Los Angeles) told a reporter.[16] A pervasive attitude throughout the United States called for not-for-profits who put themselves on the block to sell to "ABC," which stood for "anybody but Columbia."

A New Strategy

As it became more difficult for Columbia to acquire not-for-profit hospitals, it stepped outside its previous strategy by announcing plans to acquire Blue Cross and Blue Shield of Ohio. The objective was to gain more than 400,000 BC/BS members for Columbia's recently acquired hospitals in Cleveland and eventually entice other Ohio hospitals to affiliate with Columbia as they sought to hold or gain contracts with Blue Cross.

While investors remembered only Humana's fateful attempt in the late 1980s to consolidate hospitals and HMOs, Scott believed that doctors who had resisted the cost-cutting efforts of

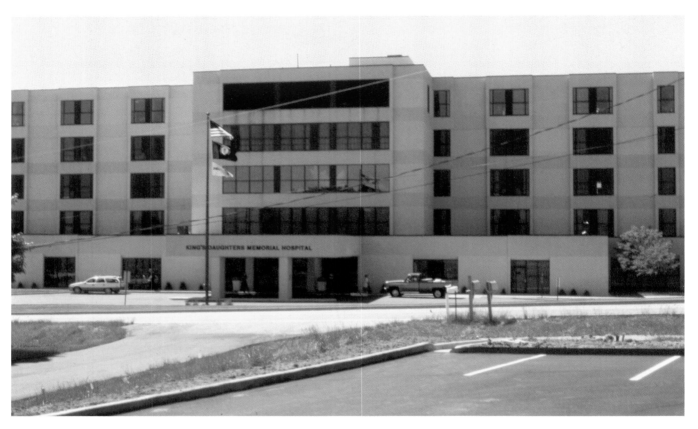

On June 6, 1994, Columbia/HCA's 190-bed King's Daughters
Memorial Hospital in Frankfort, Kentucky, was renamed Columbia
Frankfort Regional Medical Center.

HMOs led to the Humana failure. Now that health maintenance organizations were much more dominant, he believed that a hospital company–insurance company partnership made "strategic sense," especially given Blue Cross Ohio's domination of the insurance market.

The deal whipped up a firestorm of opposition and litigation. Consumer advocates insisted that the Ohio Blues' surplus reserves were accumulated with help from tax breaks and that part of it belonged to taxpayers. Meanwhile, the national association governing the nation's 63 Blue Cross and Blue Shield plans threatened to revoke the Ohio affiliate's license if it proceeded with the transaction. Policyholders approved the transaction, but in March 1997, Ohio's Department of Insurance vetoed it "as unfair and unreasonable" and "not in the public interest."[17]

National Branding

A television advertising campaign mounted by Columbia in the summer of 1996 coincided with a new era of investigative journalism. The company spent $85 million in 1995 and $106 million in 1996 on locally directed advertising, running ads during such popular shows as *Monday Night Football, Seinfeld,* and *Friends.*

As with many of Scott's decisions, there was shrewdness and logic to this one. In the world of managed care, patients had to pick a single primary care doctor from long lists—and often didn't have a clue about who the physicians were. A reasonable question for discriminating one from another might be, "If I have to go to the hospital, I want a Columbia hospital. Can the doctor get me in there?" Scott hoped that by advertising the benefits of Columbia hospitals, customers and doctors would come his way.[18]

Scott believed that healthcare was going to become more and more consumer driven and that Columbia could become the branded name of healthcare. In hindsight, the thought of corporate medicine, which the branding of Columbia implied, was unappealing to many people.[19]

Coinciding with the company's branding campaign, television had adapted to the in-your-face style of reporting that mixed entertainment with information. That fall, CBS's *60 Minutes* aired a segment on an especially controversial aspect of the proposed Ohio BC/BS acquisition: the $17 million in fees to be paid to certain Blues board members.[20]

In addition, almost everyone who had worked at HCA before the merger agreed that the culture of the new company changed dramatically after the merger with Columbia. "Culturally, HCA was very different from Columbia," noted Milton Johnson, who joined HCA in 1982, became part of HealthTrust in 1987, and later became HCA's senior vice president and chief accounting officer. "HCA was a demanding environment to work in—you had to perform—but it was a caring environment where you formed relationships with people and had mutual respect and trust. When I came into Columbia, it was a faster-paced environment. It was dynamic and exciting, but it was more competitive."[21]

By the end of 1996, Frist Jr. was cautioning Scott that he was growing too fast, not taking time to build the necessary infrastructure, making the company a lightning rod for government and public scrutiny, and working company executives too hard. Frist Jr. thought the Columbia culture treated its employees as expendable commodities. Furthermore, he was concerned about Scott's strategy of syndicating hospitals to physicians and his threatening, win-lose approach in pursuit of not-for-profits. "He just wouldn't listen," Dr. Frist Jr. recalled, more in sorrow than in anger.[22]

Clayton McWhorter saw the signs and portents. The former Columbia/HCA chairman talked with Scott in private about his concerns with the way Columbia was angering the media, the competition, and perhaps most dangerously of all, federal and state government officials.[23]

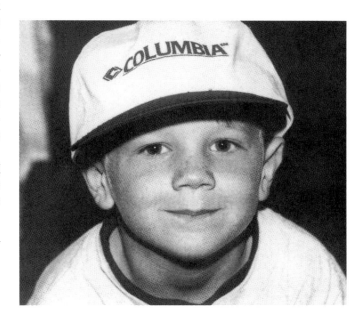

The branding campaign that Rick Scott instituted was one of many aspects of Columbia/HCA that Dr. Frist Jr. wanted to change.

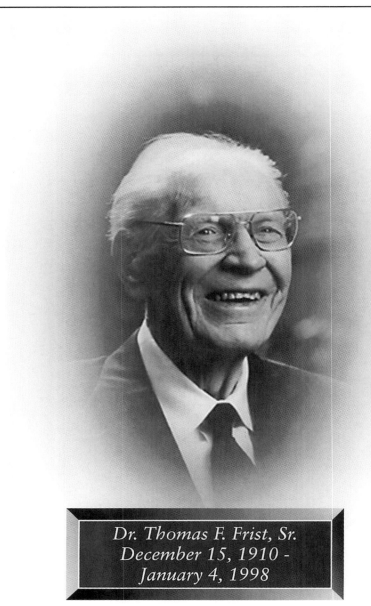

In Memory

This year, we mourn the loss and celebrate the life of Dr. Thomas F. Frist, Sr. one of the founders of Hospital Corporation of America.

A skilled physician, dedicated teacher, accomplished entrepreneur, loving family man and friend, Dr. Frist Sr. epitomized the virtues of justice, mercy and humility.

He created a record of achievement and a legacy of service that represents the best of both the American spirit and the American dream. It was upon his philosophy – "Good people beget good people," – that the foundation of this company was based.

It is his vision that we strive to perpetuate at Columbia/HCA Healthcare Corporation.

Dr. Thomas F. Frist, Sr.
December 15, 1910 -
January 4, 1998

This epitaph to Dr. Thomas Frist Sr., who died on January 4, 1998, was included with Columbia/HCA's 1997 annual report.

CHAPTER NINE

A PAINFUL ORDEAL

1997

To say that 1997 was a year of challenge is a vast understatement.

—Thomas Frist Jr., 1997

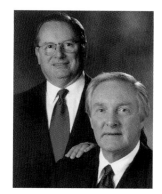

WITH THE END OF THE COLD War, many FBI agents who had previously been assigned to national security activities began instead to actively investigate Medicare reimbursement and the possibility of fraud. Across the nation, doctors, hospitals, and other recipients of Medicare reimbursement became targets of the government's scrutiny.

Hearings in Congress began to put a cloud over the hospital industry. In the winter of 1996, an investigations subcommittee of the U.S. Senate's Committee on Governmental Affairs had probed improper Medicare claims by hospitals nationwide. In February 1997, the same panel took up the subject of "Medicare at risk: emerging fraud in Medicare programs."[1]

As the largest investor-owned hospital corporation, Columbia had some critics in Congress, and its high-profile branding campaign drew the government's attention like a big neon sign. Furthermore, by targeting the largest public hospital company, the government was able to send a signal to other healthcare providers, warning them to take special care when interpreting Medicare's complicated rules and regulations.

El Paso

Suspecting Columbia of improper physician relations, the government had compiled enough

documentation against Columbia by the spring of 1997 to present a judge with probable cause that a crime or crimes had been committed. On March 19, 1997, agents from the Federal Bureau of Investigation (FBI), the U.S. Department of Health and Human Services, and the Internal Revenue Service served search warrants on the company's operations in El Paso, Texas. They also searched the offices of more than two dozen doctors.[2]

The warrants were served on the opening day of the company's annual meeting and leadership conference in Washington, D.C. Most of Columbia's management was headed to D.C. at the moment the FBI and others were sliding the warrants across the desks of startled physicians and administrators. Ironically, Columbia was in the capital to lobby Congress on legislative and regulatory matters but instead got a message about Washington's deep suspicions concerning its business dealings of recent years.[3]

"At the time, the company was flying high," remembered Jim Fitzgerald. "Our stock was at an all-time high. Everything seemed to be going great. Then someone announced that the government

Jack Bovender (left) and Dr. Thomas Frist Jr. (right) returned to the company in the summer of 1997.

was raiding our hospitals in El Paso. It was one of the most staggering, sobering moments I have ever experienced. And it was incredibly difficult for Tommy [Frist Jr.]. You could see the pain he was in."[4]

The El Paso raids were followed by two days of decline in the value of Columbia stock—from $43 a share to $38. The decline was relatively small, for it appeared that the government's issues were confined to El Paso.

Meanwhile, at the close of Columbia's meeting in Washington, Rick Scott, beset with specu-

lation and unanswered questions in the media, galvanized the audience by quoting Abraham Lincoln: "I do the very best I can," he said. Then his voice broke from emotion, and he turned and walked away.[5]

Whistleblower Lawsuits

The Justice Department's case against Columbia had taken root through civil lawsuits known as "whistleblower," or *qui tam*, suits.

Qui tam lawsuits are filed (often by employees or former employees) under a law dating back to the Civil War. Rarely used until the 1980s, whistleblower suits were revived when people who suspected fraud in government military procurement used the suits to win settlements from government contractors. Beginning in the late 1980s, the number of such suits against healthcare concerns doing business with the federal government grew rapidly.

After filing such a suit, a whistleblower forwards the case to government officials, who investigate to see whether they will join the suit. If so, the case sometimes grows into a civil or criminal investigation. The government attempts to negotiate a settlement, and the whistleblower receives a portion of any fine.[6]

A whistleblower suit against Columbia involving physician relationships had led to the El Paso raids. Another whistleblower suit charged misrepresentation of Medicare cost reports filed by HCA and HealthTrust. This suit was filed by a financial officer at North Valley Hospital in Whitefish, Montana. The hospital was managed by Quorum, a hospital company whose former financial officer had questions about the way Quorum was filing its cost reports.[7] Because HCA had once managed Quorum's hospitals, the

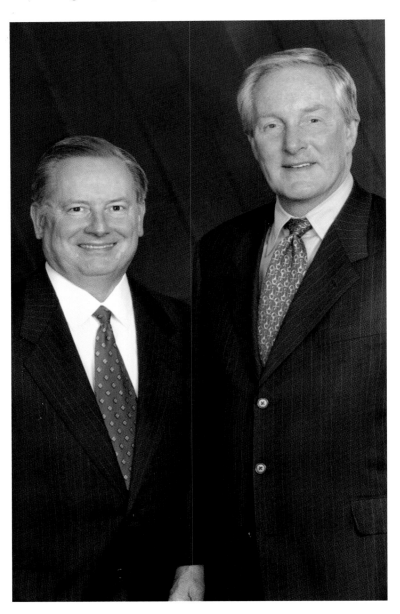

Jack Bovender (left) and Thomas Frist Jr. faced seemingly insurmountable challenges when they took over the management of Columbia/HCA. In only a few years, however, they—along with a team of dedicated executives, directors, employees, and doctors—managed to rejuvenate the company and renew the public's faith in HCA, not as a chain of hospitals but as a company devoted to healthcare.

financial officer alleged that HCA and its spin-off company, HealthTrust, might also have issues with their cost reports. Other whistleblower suits charged Medicare DRG upcoding and over-billing Medicare for home healthcare services and lab services.

Frayed Relations

Meantime, relations between Rick Scott and Dr. Frist Jr. had grown increasingly chilly. In April 1997, Frist Jr. composed a 10-page memo to Scott, which he headed, "A Proposed Revised Three to Five Year Strategic Direction." Frist Jr. prefaced the proposal with a personal note to Scott.

Dear Rick:

The Columbia story, beginning in 1987 up to this very moment, is truly remarkable. An amazing group of assets has been assembled in an unbelievably short period of time without a major misstep and, in fact, many good things have been accomplished. As a result, it is my belief that both our shareholders and our customers will be well served if we move from a growth emphasis to an operational emphasis for the next two to three years. . . . By the year 2002, Columbia/HCA, and you as its CEO, have the opportunity to earn the respect and admiration of all. . . . While not necessarily easy, if the right strategy and execution occur, my wishes for Columbia and you personally are quite realizable from the vantage point you now enjoy.

In his proposal, Frist Jr. urged Scott to, among other things, stop the branding campaign, quit the joint ventures with doctors, limit acquisitions of not-for-profit hospitals for two to three years, and shift the company to an operational phase from a growth phase. He concluded the proposal by writing, "Having expressed my thoughts to you, I stand ready to help you not only transition through this difficult period, but going forward over the coming years."

Dr. Frist Jr., an HCA founder, former executive, and huge shareholder, received not even an acknowledgment.

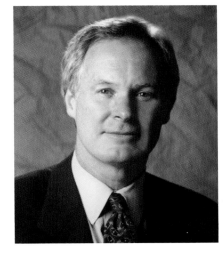

Richard Bracken began his HCA career in 1981 as CEO of a California hospital and later became a division and group president and COO. In 2002, he was named HCA president.

"I didn't know what to do," Frist Jr. told a reporter. "It was the most perplexing thing in my career."[8]

On July 16, 1997, the final shoe fell. On that day, federal agents seized Columbia documents in six states. Twenty search warrants were served in Florida, and facilities in North Carolina, Oklahoma, Tennessee, Texas, and Utah were also served.

The news sent Columbia stock plummeting 12 percent, from $38.93 a share to $34.25.[9] On CNN's *Moneyline* that evening, Scott said, "It has not been a fun day. But as you know, government investigations are matter-of-fact in healthcare." It was an accurate statement, but dismissive.[10]

Three days after the probes spread to seven states, Columbia's directors met without Scott and gave Dr. Frist Jr., Clayton McWhorter, and Michael Long, a director and partner at Brown Brothers Harriman and Company, the job of encouraging Scott to step down. In the meantime, Darla Moore, a former director, had spoken with Scott on the morning of July 17 and told him, "Rick, it's over." Perhaps all were too subtle, however. Scott insisted he could weather the storm.[11]

The directors of the embattled company convened in Nashville late in the afternoon of July 24. The meeting dragged on for hours and reconvened the next morning. On July 25, 1997, Columbia issued a press release announcing that Scott and David Vandewater, president and COO, had resigned their positions and that the board had elected Dr. Thomas Frist Jr. to succeed Scott as chairman and chief executive officer.[12] Three years later, when the restoration of the company was nearly complete, Frist Jr. told *Business Nashville* magazine that he had returned to the company to try to restore it to its position of leadership in the industry. But, he added, "I also felt a close moral obligation and commitment to those 70 hospitals that my father and I promised to be good stewards of."[13]

Right: Veteran leaders were key to Dr. Frist Jr.'s plan to rebuild HCA. Several returned to the company, such as Noel Williams (left), chief information officer, and Trish Lindler (middle), senior vice president of government programs. Other longtime executives, such as Milton Johnson (right), senior vice president and chief accounting officer, were promoted to senior positions. Williams had joined HCA in 1979 and Lindler in 1975. Both had left at the time of the Columbia merger. Johnson had joined HCA in 1982, then moved to HealthTrust in 1987, and rejoined HCA with the HealthTrust merger in 1995.

Below: Even while the company worked out its problems with the government, it continued to improve operations through a number of initiatives and reaffirmed its commitment to putting the patient "above all else."

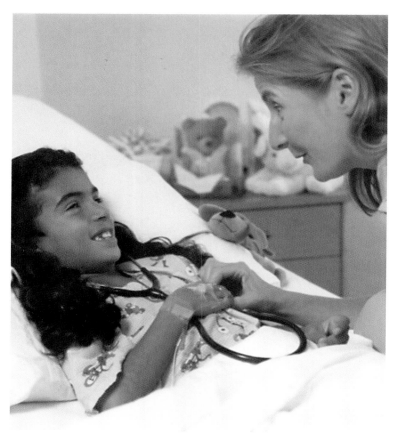

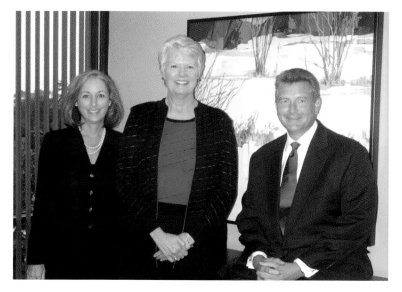

A Difficult Transition

The renaissance of a great American corporation would follow, but first certain difficulties had to be endured. Bob Waterman, whom Frist Jr. brought on in July 1997 to be HCA's lead outside counsel for the investigation (three months later, he was hired as general counsel), advised the CEO against an adversarial approach to the government, saying he thought "the government was prepared to drive the company over a cliff—and they were fully capable of doing that."[14]

Still, the management changes, the renewal of the company's values, and its wholehearted cooperation with the Justice Department did little to slow the investigation juggernaut.

Analysts pointed to the prospect of heavy fines. Yet the word on Wall Street, by and large, was "Wait and see." The company's value had proved resilient through crises before. By winter of 1998, some investors were viewing the healthcare business as "a trove of beaten-up, underpriced assets."[15]

Although a jury in Florida found two mid-level employees guilty in July 1999 of Medicare billing issues, in March 2002 the 11th U.S. Circuit Court of Appeals overruled the verdict, saying that reasonable people's interpretations could differ. "Competing interpretations of the [Medicare rules] are far too reasonable to justify these convictions," the court said.[16] The appellate court's favorable ruling was hugely significant to HCA and to the healthcare industry in general.

On May 18, 2000, Columbia announced that it had reached an agreement with the U.S. Justice Department for $745 million ($498 million after taxes) to settle certain civil fraud allegations. The agreement covered coding, outpatient laboratory billings, and home healthcare billings.

"It was a reasonable and fair settlement, and those who negotiated it were reasonable and fair people," said HCA General Counsel Bob Waterman, who led HCA's negotiating team while the terms of the settlement were being hammered out. "At the time we thought it was taking forever, but now [nearly a year later], in the cool light of day, it was a lot for the government to organize. Were they tough in negotiations? Yes. Were we tough in negotiations? Yes."[17]

Both sides had compromised to reach the agreement. The company gave up its demand that a settlement would release the company and executives from criminal charges. At the same time, the company admitted no wrongdoing and made the civil agreement contingent upon reaching a criminal settlement with the Justice Department by year's end.

On December 14, 2000, two weeks short of the deadline, the government's criminal case against Columbia was concluded. The company agreed that two of its subsidiaries would plead guilty to several counts of criminal conduct, including conspiracy. The company would also pay the federal government $95 million in penalties and fines relating to the criminal probe.[18]

Two years later, on December 18, 2002, HCA settled with the Justice Department on the remaining outstanding issues regarding cost reports and physician relations, agreeing to pay $631 million. The final settlement payment was made in July 2003, ending the Justice Department's investigation of the company.[19]

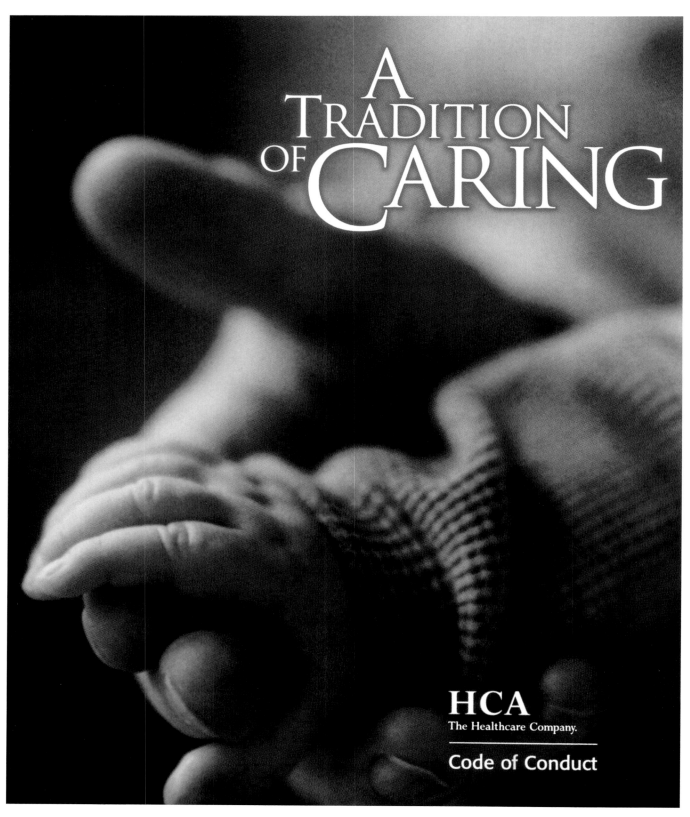

A
TRADITION
OF CARING

HCA
The Healthcare Company.

Code of Conduct

In 2000 HCA published, in brochure form, its Code of Conduct, which provided guidance to all HCA employees and doctors and was a critical component of its Ethics and Compliance program.

CHAPTER TEN

RENAISSANCE OF A HEALTHCARE COMPANY

1997–2003

Above all else, we are committed to the care and improvement of human life. In recognition of this commitment, we strive to deliver high quality, cost effective healthcare in the communities we serve.

—from the mission and values statement of HCA

ONE OF DR. FRIST JR.'S FIRST decisions upon his return to HCA proved to be the best one he could have made for the company's future: to bring back Jack Bovender as president and chief operating officer. "That was my first move, within the first 24 hours," said Frist Jr. "[Bovender] lives and breathes the values that I hold dear and that I think this corporate institution should embrace."[1]

Frist Jr. and Bovender made another important decision upon their return to the company. Richard Bracken, who had recently resigned as Columbia's president of the Pacific Division, returned to HCA as president of the Western Group.

Bracken had joined HCA in 1981 as an assistant administrator in one of the company's California hospitals and was shortly promoted to CEO for a hospital in the Los Angeles area. Over the years, he served as CEO of several HCA hospitals—including Scripps Clinic and Research Foundation in La Jolla and Centennial Medical Center in Nashville—before becoming president of the Pacific Division in 1995.

Bracken, who would later be named HCA's president, initially would be responsible for half of the company's hospital operations, those west of the Mississippi River. Jay Grinney, one of Columbia's five group presidents, would be responsible for the other half, those east of the Mississippi.

Frist Jr. and Bovender laid their shoulders to the wheel to resolve the investigations and to renew the company's commitment to the care and improvement of human life. Symbolic of this rebirth, in 2000 the company dropped the word Columbia from its name and became once again HCA, or to many, Hospital Corporation of America.

Michael Watras, owner of the firm HCA had hired to help rename itself, said that he'd never worked with a company that chose to go back to its previous name. "But again," he said, "it was probably the first time in my 20 years of working on projects like this where so many people supported the fact that HCA had been a great company... and that HCA was a great name."[2] Or, as Frist Jr. and Bovender pointed out, "Returning the company's name to HCA is an affirmation of the culture and values of our ... employees."[3]

The HCA Foundation, which funds programs in middle Tennessee and southern Kentucky, supports health and wellness, childhood development, and quality of life. Shown here is a young patient wondering how much he weighs.

Above all else, we are committed to the care and improvement of human life. In recognition of this commitment, we strive to deliver high quality, cost effective healthcare in the communities we serve.

Frist Jr. and Bovender began the renaissance of the company with what they called a 12-point action plan, rolled out on August 7, 1997, less than two weeks after Frist Jr. returned as chairman and CEO. The 12-point plan included a wide range of initiatives.

Above: The company's new mission and values statement was a result of input from more than 10,000 employees and physicians. It was published on the cover of the 1997 annual report. The mission statement (pictured) filled the front cover, and the values statement appeared on the report's back cover.

Left: This bronze statue is presented annually to winners of the Frist Humanitarian Award, which recognizes employees and volunteers in HCA hospitals "who daily perform their work with concern, in a spirit of love, and with humility and understanding."

Succinctly put, the 12-point plan proposed the following:

- *New leadership*
- *Internal audit of policies and procedures*
- *Institutionalization of a values-based culture*
- *Development of a model compliance program*
- *Elimination of short-term cash bonuses*
- *Return to local community focus*
- *Divestiture of home healthcare operations*
- *Implementation of an OIG lab compliance program*
- *Provision for a second review of certain DRG codes*
- *An increase in cost-report disclosure*
- *An end to the establishment of physician syndications of hospitals*
- *Increased security of physician transactions*

Later, Dr. Frist Jr. acknowledged that he was surprised by what turned out to be the major challenges behind HCA's renaissance. "Jack and I returned thinking that solving the fraud and abuse issues was the primary challenge, but we quickly learned we had a company that was operationally out of control," Frist Jr. said. "If the federal government had not caused a change in management, I believe Columbia would have imploded within six months, not unlike Enron and WorldCom several years later."

Mission and Values

Perhaps the most critical piece of the 12-point plan was fostering a values-based culture, for this was a concept to which each of the company's more than 160,000 employees must adhere.

On October 24, 1997, Frist Jr. and Bovender flew out of Nashville on their first extended tour of company hospitals since returning. For the next two months, they rode the circuit from Plano, Texas, to Richmond, Virginia, and many points between. They carried with them a white banner—the company's new mission and values statement—which local management helped drape across the auditoriums where they spoke. Frist Jr. and Bovender invited employees to sign this new declaration of purpose with them. They whisked their magic marker at the bottom of the text, and listeners stepped forward to add their names.[4]

"Above all else, we are committed to the care and improvement of human life," the new mission and values statement read. It continued:

In recognition of this commitment, we strive to deliver high quality, cost effective healthcare in the communities we serve.

In pursuit of our mission, we believe the following value statements are essential and timeless.

- *We recognize and affirm the unique and intrinsic worth of each individual.*
- *We treat all those we serve with compassion and kindness.*
- *We act with absolute honesty, integrity, and fairness in the way we conduct our business and the way we live our lives.*
- *We trust our colleagues as valuable members of our healthcare team and pledge to treat one another with loyalty, respect, and dignity.*

Frist Jr. and Bovender had invited focus groups of thousands of employees throughout the country to create the new mission and values statement, which contained not a single word about financial performance. Dr. Frist Sr. had advised, years before, to take care of the patient—and the bottom line would take care of itself. HCA had not forgotten his wisdom. Three years later, Frist Jr. told a Nashville business reporter that developing the mission and values statement was the single most important thing he and Bovender did in restoring the company. "Yet that would have been a wasteful exercise if, in fact, everything we do in our corporate lives ... doesn't reinforce that statement. You live and breathe it."[5]

HCA backed the words of its new creed with action, putting into place a division of Ethics and Compliance and hiring Alan R. Yuspeh as senior vice president for ethics, compliance, and corporate responsibility. Yuspeh had earned his spurs establishing programs for the defense industry, and Dr. Frist Jr. wanted him to set up the best compliance program ever established in American business. Beginning in 1998, every employee of the company heard an hour-long presentation of its new Code of Conduct, "One Clear Voice." Employees were encouraged to raise concerns—to be "obtrusive and repetitive"—and the company provided a 1-800 Ethics Line. Dr. Frist Jr. wrote thank-you notes to employees who brought problems to their supervisors' attention.[6]

"What we've found throughout the organization is people desperately want to do the right thing," he told a business conference three years into the program.[7]

Frist Jr. and Bovender also promoted Dr. Frank Houser to medical director and senior vice president of quality. Dr. Houser would oversee outcomes measurement, benchmarking, and standards assessment; patient and physician satisfaction; education, training, and new technology; and best demonstrated processes.

Making Repairs

Most of the directives in the 12-point plan were concrete and saw near-immediate resolution. To keep the company's focus on long-term development of quality care, hospital CEOs would no longer receive an annual cash incentive. This measure broke the connection between paychecks and short-term objectives. And no longer would HCA sell hospital interests to physicians.

The management team carefully reviewed and strengthened its policies and procedures for DRG coding and other gray areas of Medicare reimbursement.

A Local Community Focus

HCA's management team had also committed to returning to a local community focus. "Healthcare is very local in certain respects," explained Bracken. "The relationships with the physicians, the community, and the employee base—these are not things that can be orchestrated from Nashville."[8]

Management promised more responsiveness—and less control—from the corporate office. Local hospitals were given more decision-making power. "We [at corporate] make sure we have a strategic plan for how we're going to take care of the needs of communities, but the actual decisions have to be figured out locally," said Bovender. He went on to add that it was corporate's job to "make sure our hospitals are built around the concept of having the best and brightest doctors in the community practicing there, that we recruit the best employees to work there, and that we are oriented toward pro-

viding good care for patients and patients' families. But the decisions have to be made locally."[9] This was a company tradition that went back to Dr. Frist Sr.—that people nearest the problems could be relied upon to provide quality medical care and honesty in business dealings.

Even before Bovender reported for duty, Frist Jr. had pulled the plug on the national branding campaign. The new management team told local hospitals and networks they were free to drop Columbia from their names and develop name identities that made sense from a local community standpoint.[10]

Part of the return to local focus meant working more cooperatively with others in the health-care industry. HCA canceled eight construction projects that were perceived as "in your face" competition with not-for-profits and sold a number of its hospitals to not-for-profit buyers.

Operations Focus

Frist Jr. and Bovender believed that Columbia had become too large in terms of hospital numbers and too diverse in the healthcare businesses it managed. "We had a lot of problems," said Bovender, "and many of them came from Columbia's aggressive acquisition strategy. There had been five companies essentially jammed together in a very short time. We needed to change from an acquisitions-oriented company to an operations-oriented one."[11]

Unlike HCA during its successful rapid growth phase in the 1980s, Columbia had no long-standing corporate culture and operating infrastructure, so it was difficult to successfully assimilate the various hospitals it had acquired into one organization. HCA had been disciplined enough to sell assets and change management that did not fit the corporate culture, and now it began asserting that discipline once again.

In November 1997, the two leaders announced an internal operating reorganization that would create smaller, more independent, community-based hospital groups. This restructuring, Frist Jr.

Opposite: In its 1999 annual report, HCA pledged to "keep an eye on what matters most—our patients."

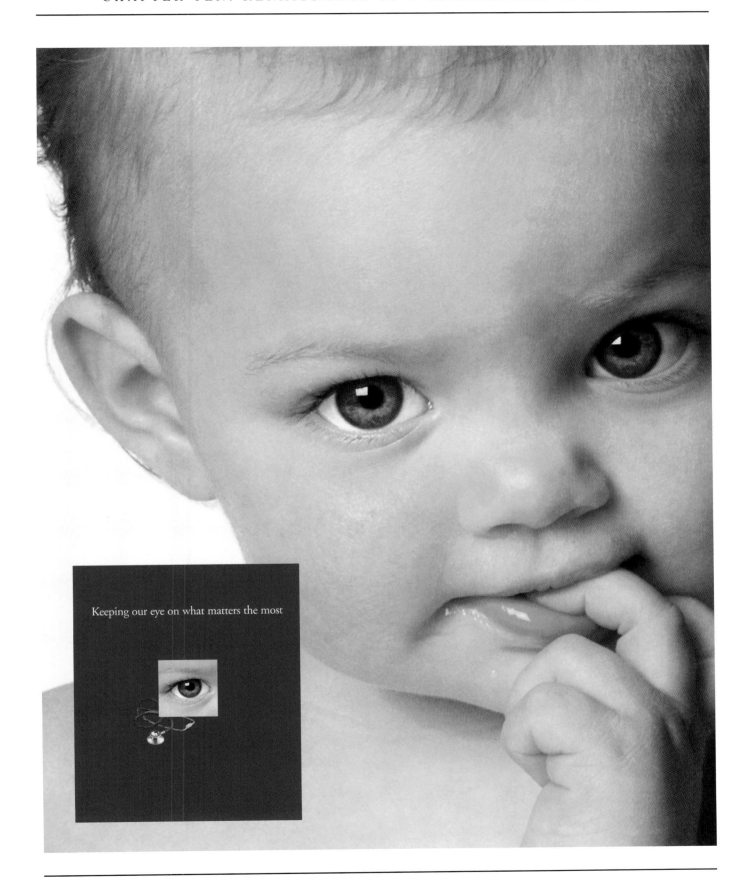

Keeping our eye on what matters the most

CHANGE AT THE TOP

DR. FRIST JR. AND JACK BOVENDER agreed that HCA could "only be as good as the people who are running the place."[1] Almost overnight, a company with $20 billion in revenue and 280,000 employees removed the majority of its top 12 senior managers and set about building a top-notch management team. (At the same time, Dr. Frist Jr. began assembling a world-class board of directors comparable to HCA's board in the 1980s.) Beginning in the summer of 1997, many HCA officers were elevated to more senior positions, and others were brought in from the outside. By 2003 HCA's preeminent management team was a melting pot of HCA veterans and new hires.

The Leaders

Thomas Frist Jr., M.D., HCA cofounder. Frist Jr. cofounded HCA in 1968 and has since served the company in a variety of leadership positions, including executive vice president, chief operating officer, president, chief executive officer, and chairman of the board. He retired from active duty in 2001, serving HCA in his retirement as a board member.

Jack O. Bovender Jr., chairman and CEO. Bovender began his hospital administrative career in 1969 as a lieutenant in the U.S. Navy. He went on to become CEO of two HCA hospitals: Medical Center Hospital in Largo, Florida, and West Florida Regional Medical Center in Pensacola. Bovender held several senior-level positions at HCA from 1985 to 1992, when he was named executive vice president and COO of HCA. He left the company in 1994 and returned in 1997 as president and COO. He was named president and CEO in 2001 and became chairman and CEO in January 2002.

Richard M. Bracken, president and COO. Bracken began his HCA career in 1981, holding various executive positions, including CEO of the Green Hospital of Scripps Clinic and Research Foundation in San Diego and CEO of Centennial Medical Center in Nashville. Bracken became president of the Pacific Division in 1995 and president of the Western Group in 1997. He was promoted to COO in July 2001 and to president and COO in January 2002.

The Senior Vice Presidents

David G. Anderson, senior vice president, finance and treasurer. Anderson began his career in 1978 as a manager of finance at Humana. In 1993 he became vice president of finance and treasurer of Galen Health Care, a spin-off of Humana that was later acquired by HCA. He was promoted to senior vice president, finance and treasurer in July 1998.

Victor L. Campbell, senior vice president. Campbell joined HCA's finance department in 1972 and established the company's investor relations function in 1976. He was named senior vice president, investor relations, in 1994 and is also responsible for government relations and communications. Campbell is HCA's primary liaison with the AHA and FAH.

Rosalyn S. Elton, senior vice president, operations finance. Elton joined Columbia in 1988 and was named vice president of operations finance in 1999. She was promoted to senior vice president in 1999 and is responsible for planning HCA's capital and operating budgets, analyzing the financial operations of company hospitals, and managing the process of allocating $2 billion each year to reinvest in HCA's facilities.

James A. Fitzgerald Jr., senior vice president, contracts and operations support. Fitzgerald joined HCA in 1981 as director of internal audit and held several other positions before becoming assistant vice president of operations support in 1993 and vice president of contracts and operations support in 1994. He was promoted to his current position in 1999 and is responsible for managing HCA's supply chain services initiative.

V. Carl George, senior vice president, development. George joined HCA in 1969 as assistant treasurer and has served in a variety of positions, including assistant vice president of finance for HCA's former Australian subsidiary. In 1987 he joined HealthTrust, an HCA spin-off company, as director of development. George returned to HCA in 1995, when HCA reacquired HealthTrust, and was promoted to vice president of development in 1997. He has served in his current position since 1999.

Jay Grinney, president – Eastern Group. Grinney joined Columbia in 1990 as CEO of Rosewood Medical Center in Houston. He became COO of Columbia's Houston Region in 1992 and president of the Greater Houston Division in 1993. He was named a group president in 1996 and rose to his current position in 1998.

Samuel N. Hazen, president – Western Group. Hazen began his career in Humana's Financial Management Training Program in 1983 and served as CFO for several hospitals before joining HCA in 1994 as CFO of the North Texas Division. He became CFO of the Western Group in 1995 and was promoted to his current position in July 2001.

Frank M. Houser, M.D., senior vice president, quality and medical director. Houser began his career in 1971 as a pediatrician at the Pediatric Clinic of Dalton in Dalton, Georgia. He served in various positions in the state's healthcare department before he was appointed Georgia's state director of public health in 1991. Houser joined Columbia/HCA in 1994 as president of the Georgia Division. He became president of HCA Physician Services in 1996 and began his current position in 1997.

R. Milton Johnson, senior vice president, controller, and chief accounting officer. Johnson joined HCA in 1982 as tax manager in the research and planning area and later became director of tax for HealthTrust, an HCA spin-off company. He returned to HCA as vice president of tax in 1995, when HCA reacquired HealthTrust, and was named to his current position in 1999.

Patricia T. Lindler, senior vice president, government programs. Lindler joined HCA in 1975 as an internal auditor and has since held various reimbursement positions, including director of reimbursement for HCA's Florida Group operations. She left HCA in 1995 to become president of Health Financial Directions and returned to HCA in 1998 as vice president of reimbursement. She has held her current position since 1999.

A. Bruce Moore Jr., senior vice president, operations administration. Moore joined HCA in 1982 as a staff auditor and has held a variety of positions, including vice president of compensation and vice president of benefits, before becoming vice president of operations administration in 1997. He has served in his current position since 1999.

Philip R. Patton, senior vice president, human resources. Patton joined HCA in 1979 and served as senior vice president of human resources from 1992 to 1994. He then went to Quorum Health Group as vice president for human resources. In 1998 he rejoined HCA in his current role. In addition to overseeing HCA's human resources, Patton has administrative oversight for Corporate Services, the HCA Foundation, and Community Outreach.

Gregory S. Roth, president – Ambulatory Surgery Group. Roth joined Columbia/HCA in 1995 as CFO of the Ambulatory Surgery Division. He became senior vice president of the Western Region of the Ambulatory Surgery Division in 1997 and president of the Ambulatory Surgery Group in 1998. He was named a senior vice president in 1999.

William B. Rutherford, chief financial officer – Eastern Group. Rutherford began his HCA career in 1986 and has served in several positions, including director of internal audit, director of operations support, and CFO of the Georgia Division. He has been in his current role since 1996.

Richard J. Shallcross, chief financial officer – Western Group. Shallcross was CFO of Rose Healthcare System in Denver when HCA acquired it in 1995. He then became vice president of finance and managed care for HCA's Colorado Division and in 1996 became CFO of the Utah/Idaho Division. In 1997 Shallcross became CFO of the Continental Division. He has served in his current position since 2001.

Joseph N. Steakley, senior vice president, internal audit and consulting services. Steakley joined HCA in 1997 as vice president of internal audit and consulting services and was promoted to senior vice president in 1999. Previously he had been a partner at Ernst & Young, where he worked for 22 years.

Beverly B. Wallace, president, financial services. Wallace began her career with Humana in 1983 as CFO at the hospital, market, and division level in the company's hospital operations, which was renamed Galen. She joined HCA in 1993 when HCA purchased Galen and served as CFO for the Nashville and Mid-Atlantic divisions. In 1998 Wallace was appointed vice president of managed care and was named to her current position in 1999.

Robert A. Waterman, senior vice president and general counsel. Waterman joined HCA in late 1997 in his current position. Waterman initially came into the company in the summer of 1997 as part of a team from Latham & Watkins, which HCA hired to help resolve the government investigation. Late that year, he became senior vice president and general counsel.

Noel Brown Williams, senior vice president, chief information officer, and president of HCA information technology and services. Williams joined HCA in 1979 and spent 13 years in HCA's information services department in a variety of positions, including vice president of information services from 1994 to 1995. She left HCA in 1995 to become chief information officer for America Service Group in Brentwood, Tennessee, and rejoined HCA in 1997 in her current position.

Alan R. Yuspeh, senior vice president, ethics, compliance, and corporate responsibility. Yuspeh, a nationally recognized expert in corporate ethics and compliance, joined HCA in 1997 in his current position. He previously held a variety of management consultant positions. Most recently he served for 10 years as coordinator of the Defense Industry Initiative on Business Ethics and Conduct.

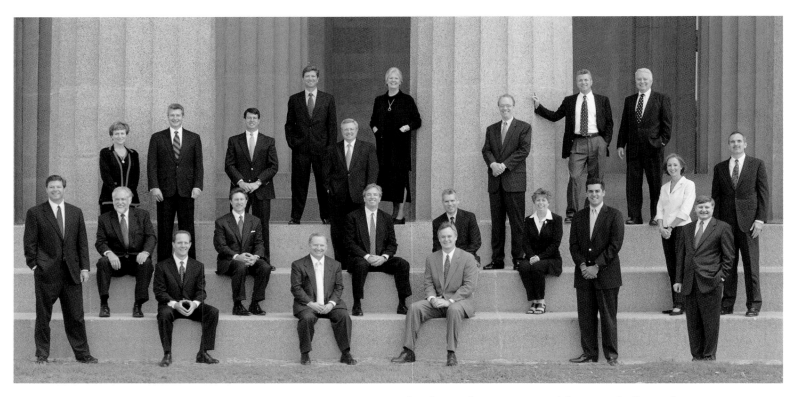

HCA's top managers gather for a 2002 photo, later presented to Dr. Frist Jr. when he stepped down as chairman. Standing on grass, from left: Bruce Moore, Sam Hazen, and Alan Yuspeh. Sitting on bottom stair, from left: Jay Grinney, Jack Bovender, and Richard Bracken. Sitting on second stair, from left: Carl George, Joseph Steakley, Vic Campbell, Bob Waterman, and Beverly Wallace. Standing on bottom stair (at right): Noel Williams and Greg Roth. Standing on second stair, from left: Ros Elton, Milton Johnson, Bill Rutherford, David Anderson, and Phil Patton. Standing on top stair, from left: James Fitzgerald, Trish Lindler, Rick Shallcross, and Frank Houser.

announced, would enhance HCA's "commitment to providing quality patient care through local hospitals and local healthcare networks."[12]

Frist Jr., Bovender, and group presidents Richard Bracken and Jay Grinney took a careful look at HCA's assets and determined that there were markets where the company clearly was not a leading provider and never would be without investing huge amounts of capital. Recognizing that capital was limited, they determined that HCA should keep only those hospitals where it was a market leader or had the potential to be a market leader within a reasonable period of time by investing a reasonable amount of capital.

"We wanted to have a strong local network, and we wanted to be in the larger urban markets," said Bracken. "We wanted to have assets that had a chance of growing and improving, and we put that filter over all our hospitals to decide which ones to divest."[13]

To better support local hospitals, HCA cut its number of divisions from 36 to 11. It divested home healthcare facilities in 24 states and sold 33 outpatient surgery centers in communities where HCA did not have a strong hospital network.

HCA's overarching goal was to downsize and focus its operations in growing urban communities where it had leading hospital networks. In early 1998, these core hospitals—roughly 200 of them—were organized into two operating groups, those east of the Mississippi (Eastern Group) and those west (Western Group). Approximately 100 hospitals were placed into three operating groups (Rural, National, and Atlantic), where they would remain until various regulatory approvals could be obtained for tax-free spin-offs to shareholders. Another 40-plus hospitals were designated for sale.

In the summer of 1998, the company received an unsolicited offer from a consortium of not-for-profits to buy the 21-hospital Atlantic Group. Although somewhat concerned that the IRS might not approve all three spin-offs (never before had any public company sought approval for more than two tax-free spins), HCA consummated the $1.2 billion sale in November 1998.

Approvals for the two remaining spin-offs were obtained by May 1999, and HCA shareholders received stock in two new public companies. LifePoint Hospitals (formerly the Rural Group) contained 23 small, rural hospitals. LifePoint would retain its corporate headquarters in Nashville under the leadership of chairman and CEO Scott Mercy, president and COO Jim Fleetwood, and CFO Ken Donahey. (All of these men were longtime HCA and/or HealthTrust executives.)

Triad Hospitals (formerly the National Group) was made up of 34 small to mid-size suburban hospitals, mostly in the West. Denny Shelton, a Columbia/HCA group president since 1994, was named chairman, CEO, and president of Triad, which would be based in Dallas.

As with the HealthTrust and Quorum spin-offs in earlier years, LifePoint and Triad employees (mostly former HCA employees) and the communities where the hospitals were located all benefited. Dr. Frist Jr. chose the management teams for both new hospital companies from among HCA's management. Under the umbrella of a smaller, strategically focused company, the hospitals could enjoy more attention from management, have more capital available, and be better able to take advantage of local market conditions and relationships. Both LifePoint and Triad proved very successful because they could tailor their strategies and operational capabilities to the defining characteristics of their hospitals.[14] Both proved to be strong, independent public companies.

Inevitably, one reporter expressed the company's reorganization strategy in a sports metaphor: HCA had "dropped a weight class and entered the ring a stronger fighter."[15] Dr. Frist Jr. put it another way. "It's about Grand Strand Medical Center in Myrtle Beach, South Carolina, and the babies born there today." This was another way of stating HCA's philosophy to make patients the first priority.

Good Returns

By 1999 Frist Jr. and Bovender had begun to see results from the new course they had charted. Despite the Balanced Budget Act (BBA) of 1997, which had reduced HCA's Medicare reimbursements for 1998 by about $215 million,[16] the company's earnings from continuing operations met or exceeded analysts' expectations, beginning in the first quarter of 1999 and continuing in subsequent quarters. Cash flow was increasing, too. At last the company was off the critical list.[17]

Other measurements showed how far the company had come: Patient satisfaction rose, according to surveys at facilities. And the company achieved what it saw as "right sizing," or "the finest portfolio of hospitals ever assembled in one organization."[18] Also, in 2001 physician satisfaction with HCA hospitals was at its highest level in five years.[19]

From 1997 to 2001 the company generated some $5 billion from divesting assets and was able to return to generating strong operating cash flow. As a result, it was able to repurchase $5 billion of common stock at deflated prices and reduce debt by almost $5 billion. At the same time, it reinvested more than $5 billion in its hospitals. Technology and new and expanded services topped the list of projects.[20] And by strengthening its hospital networks with the latest services, HCA attracted new patients, quality healthcare workers, and physicians. Furthermore, HCA ensured that it would always have a pipeline of quality employees by establishing a focused management development program.

The operational restructuring and the company's emphasis on values culminated in a truly remarkable renaissance of HCA. In tremendous solidarity, company executives expressed their joy at working for such a company and attributed HCA's revival to Dr. Frist Jr. and Bovender.

"When I was hired, people did not want to work for this company, but that's changed," said Joe Steakley, a senior vice president who was hired as head of the internal audit group in 1997, in the midst of the company's troubles. Steakley had confidence in Frist Jr.'s and Bovender's abilities to right the sinking ship. "I had known them for a number of years, and I never flinched from walking away from a pretty decent job as a partner at Ernst & Young."[21]

The story of HCA's renaissance and bright future was featured in some of the industry's leading magazines. The cover of a June 2000 *Modern Healthcare* pictured (from left) Jack Bovender, Vic Campbell, and Dr. Thomas Frist Jr. *(Reprinted with permission from* Modern Healthcare, *copyright Crain Communications Inc., 360 N. Michigan Ave., Chicago, IL 60601.)*

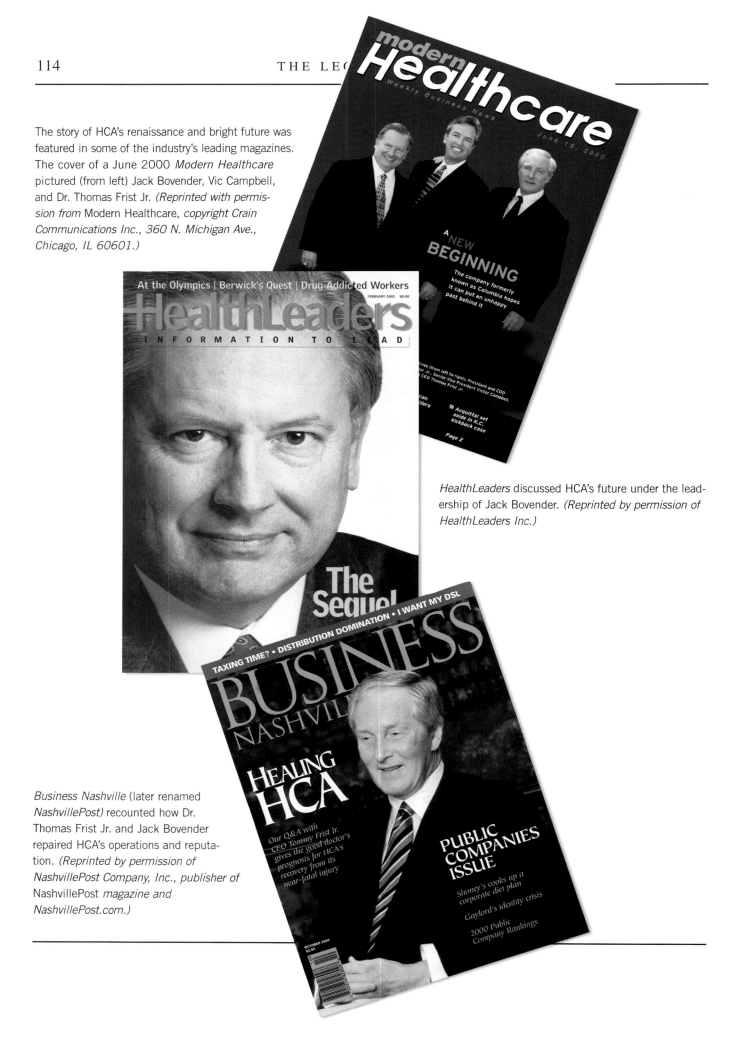

HealthLeaders discussed HCA's future under the leadership of Jack Bovender. *(Reprinted by permission of HealthLeaders Inc.)*

Business Nashville (later renamed *NashvillePost)* recounted how Dr. Thomas Frist Jr. and Jack Bovender repaired HCA's operations and reputation. *(Reprinted by permission of NashvillePost Company, Inc., publisher of* NashvillePost *magazine and* NashvillePost.com.)*

"Not many people have the leadership ability of Dr. Frist Jr. and Jack Bovender," said Bill Rutherford, CFO of HCA's Eastern Group. "The organization at the time was so complex, and with the internal and external pressures we had, they were able to envision the future, and then lay the groundwork for executing it."[22]

Reforming Medicare—Again

At the same time that HCA was addressing company-specific issues, its hospitals were beginning to feel devastating impacts from the BBA of 1997.[23]

In the late fall of 1998, HCA saw that the BBA was cutting much deeper than intended, and management was determined to take action. Frist Jr. and Vic Campbell were the first in the industry to bring the seriousness of the cuts to the attention of the American Hospital Association (AHA), which represents all U.S. hospitals; the Federation of American Hospitals (FAH), which represents investor-owned hospitals; and the Tennessee Hospital Association (THA), which represents Tennessee hospitals. From there, Dick Davidson (executive director of the AHA), Tom Scully (executive director of the FAH), and Craig Becker (president of the THA) began a concerted effort to better understand how BBA was affecting individual hospitals across the country. Davidson, Scully, and Becker, along with other state hospital association executives, led a grassroots effort to gather data on how badly BBA had overshot its original goals and how the drastic cuts could put some hospitals out of business. By early 1999, the BBA had exceeded its goal, having already cut Medicare expenditures by about $260 billion rather than Congress's intended goal of $100 billion over five years. The entire healthcare industry joined in the effort and communicated its concerns to members of Congress.[24]

The grassroots campaign paid off when Congress passed the 1999 Balanced Budget Refinement Act (BBRA), which reduced future Medicare cuts, and the 2000 Benefit Improvement and Protection Act (BIPA), which helped compensate for some of the extensive cuts that had taken place. In 2001 hospitals received their first increase in Medicare payment rates since October 1996.[25]

Managed Care Strategy

A key element in HCA's operational turnaround, along with getting the right assets in place, was developing a strategy for negotiating contracts with managed care companies, which in 1998 accounted for about 40 percent of HCA's admissions. The hospital industry had been giving substantial discounts to HMOs and other managed care companies, and Bovender was convinced that the discounts were too steep, that hospital companies were not getting a fair return.

Vic Campbell recalled Bovender coming into his office his first week back at HCA and talking about a flawed managed care strategy. "What's flawed about it?" Campbell remembered asking, and then he listened as Bovender laid out his case. HCA (and other hospitals for that matter) were offering discounts to managed care to bring in more business. But Bovender argued that HCA would have got the business whether it offered discounts or not. He suspected HCA was losing money on many managed care contracts and not getting a fair return

Skyline Medical Center on Dickerson Road in Nashville opened its doors on September 15, 2000. The $102 million hospital boasts state-of-the-art emergency service and critical-care units.

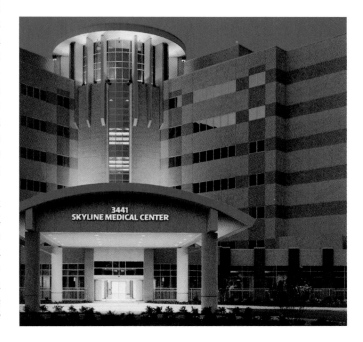

A COMMITMENT TO COMMUNITIES

HCA'S COMMITMENT TO THE CARE and improvement of human life extends beyond the walls of its hospitals and surgery centers to the greater community.

For many years, HCA had been making donations to the United Way, and that tradition continued after the September 11, 2001, terrorist attacks. Only a few days after the attacks, HCA donated $2 million to the September 11th Fund, created by the United Way and the New York Community Trust to mobilize financial resources for the victims and their families. The contribution, Bovender announced, was made on behalf of all of HCA's 170,000 employees, many of whom had been inquiring as to how they could help in the country's time of need.[1]

A few months later, in December, HCA joined with the U.S. Labor Department to create a partnership designed to combat the growing shortage of healthcare workers by training and employing people in healthcare careers. The partnership targeted people who had lost their jobs after the September 11 attacks.[2]

HCA also contributed to the country's efforts for community-based disaster readiness by adopting defined levels of preparedness at its hospitals. It provided hospital administrative and clinical leadership in community-based readiness. Other community hospitals and federal and state agencies have adopted HCA's standards for modeling of healthcare disaster preparedness programs. In addition, HCA sponsored two medical teams that the U.S. Department of Health and Human Services could mobilize in times of need.[3]

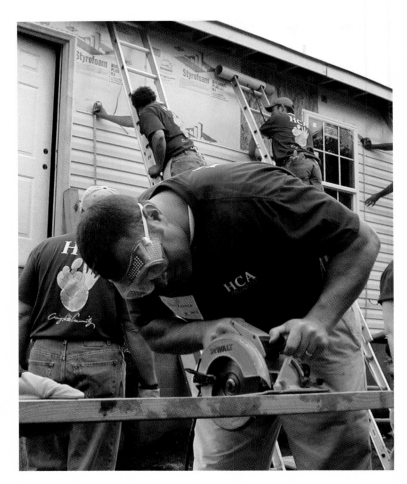

Above: Habitat for Humanity has become a favorite charity of HCA. In 2001 the company started its "Build a Hospital— Build a Home" project to fund and build a Habitat home in conjunction with building or renovating new hospitals.

Opposite: HCA has long been a supporter of United Way. Jack Bovender takes part in a 1999 United Way fundraiser race in Nashville's Centennial Park (bottom). The race included an entry "flown" by HCA Chairman Thomas Frist Jr., himself a licensed pilot (top). *(Photographs courtesy Terri Hicks.)*

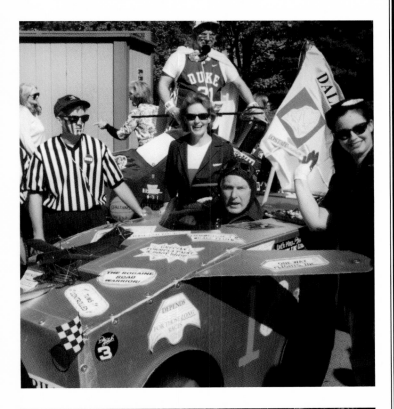

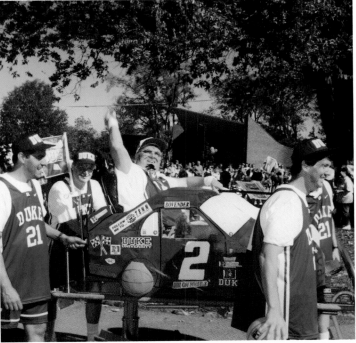

on others. That meant HCA was less able to provide services that patients wanted and deserved.

Campbell asked Bovender which contracts he was referring to. Bovender acknowledged that he hadn't studied a single contract but that he knew there was a problem just from looking at the overall picture. "We're going to figure it out," he told Campbell.[26]

Bovender appointed Beverly Wallace, senior vice president of revenue cycle operations management, to uncover the data that proved his intuition was correct. He then put a process in place to ensure that future contracts would either yield a fair return or else be terminated.

Previously HCA had been offering discounts on managed care pricing in order to generate volume. But as Bovender pointed out, Wallace's study made management realize that "more admissions at a bad price is a recipe for financial disaster." By early 1999, HCA had begun to negotiate improved prices with managed care contracts, and the new prices had a dramatic effect on the company's future.[27] Other hospitals saw what HCA was doing and realized that they, too, were discounting their prices too much. It wasn't long before they too began negotiating more favorable managed care agreements.[28] As the *Wall Street Journal* reported in April 2002, "Big insurance companies held the upper hand in the struggle over prices charged by hospitals.... In a little known power shift since the late 1990s, HCA and other major hospital chains have reshaped themselves into local oligopolists with the muscle to enforce much higher prices."[29]

HCA based its reception of managed care contracts on a baseline of acceptability that allowed for the differing needs and dynamics of each community. The company would not accept contracts that did not appropriately reimburse HCA or offer clear, concrete administrative language for adjudication of claims or straightforward processes for prompt payment and for handling denials. By 2000 HCA had used this baseline of acceptability to renegotiate nearly every one of its managed care contracts.[30]

The managed care strategy complemented HCA's operational strategy, just as HCA had intended. Owning the number one or number two hospital or hospital group in a community gave HCA better leverage in negotiations with managed care organizations than it had enjoyed with 340 hospitals scattered nationwide. And HCA was able to formulate its baseline of acceptability based on individual communities only because it had become a more focused company.[31]

In April 2002 *Business Week* reported that Bovender's managed care strategy "marked a turning point in the company's health, if not the industry's."[32]

Shared Services

Yet another piece in HCA's overall strategy was the shared services program, initiated by Milton Johnson, senior vice president and controller, and executed by Beverly Wallace and Jim Fitzgerald.

The concept of sharing administrative and business services among geographically separated entities, while very common in a lot of industries, had never been accomplished effectively in the hospital industry. Creating the infrastructure needed for shared services was expensive, and only within the past 10 years had a healthcare company been large enough or interested enough to foot the bill for such a strategy. A 20-hospital system, for example, would not be able to effectively put together the resources and infrastructure and still save enough to justify the initial expense.[33]

With HCA's assets concentrated in major markets, it was able to set up a shared services infrastructure to streamline purchasing and distribution functions as well as billing and collections.

HCA took the administrative "back office" functions of hospitals, including billing and collections, and aggregated them into 10 local centers around

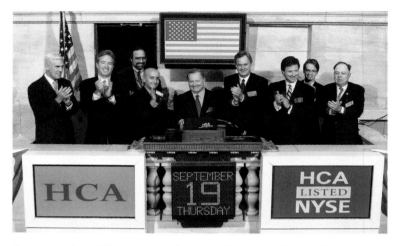

the country. This not only saved money but also allowed local hospitals to concentrate their people and other resources on improving patient care.

"This complements our managed care strategy," explained Beverly Wallace. "The people who work in the patient accounts service centers are experts in dealing with the most prevalent insurance plans for the hospitals in their network. They get to know the people at the insurance companies; they sit down and meet with them. And by processing accounts receivable more rapidly and efficiently, by eliminating that function from a hospital CEO's worry list, the accounts receivable days are dropping, and that means big savings for HCA."[34]

"We have fewer contact points," added Milton Johnson, "and that allows us to be more consistent in our contracting with managed care companies. As a result, we get paid faster and more accurately."[35]

Johnson explained another benefit of shared services. "The consolidation helps us understand

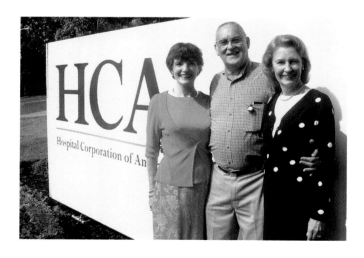

Above: In 2002 the New York Stock Exchange honored HCA by inviting the company to open the day's trading. CEO Jack Bovender (center) rings the bell while Senior Vice President Vic Campbell (second from left), President Richard Bracken (to the right of Bovender), and Mark Kimbrough (beside Bracken), vice president of investor relations, give a round of applause.

Left: Longtime HCA employees (from left) Mary Greer (34 years in 2003), Bud Reed (22 years in 2003), and Cynthia Smith (31 years in 2003) were happy to see the company return to its roots as Hospital Corporation of America.

our sources of revenue better," he said. "So in addition to taking cost out, it's allowed us to improve the overall operations of the company."[36]

Under Jim Fitzgerald's leadership, HCA also consolidated its supply procurement and warehousing into 10 centers to lower supply chain–related costs and improve productivity. "HCA's supply chain has allowed us to take control of nearly all of the procurement and distribution functions required to move supplies from the manufacturer to the end user at the hospital," said Fitzgerald. "Standardizing processes and systems has also provided much better interaction regarding new medical technologies and the utilization of supplies."[37]

The company also used its size advantage to create one of the industry's largest group purchasing organizations. Borrowing from an old name, the group purchasing organization (GPO) became

HealthTrust Purchasing Group (HPG). Originally designed to allow spin-off companies LifePoint and Triad to participate in the economies of scale enjoyed by HCA's hospitals, HPG was soon opened to other participants.

"Today HPG has over 650 hospital members and annual purchasing power of $5.5 billion," Fitzgerald said. "HPG's 'patients first' philosophy has created industry-best pricing due to its members' compliance or support for its contracts."

"We did a lot of planning on the front end before we kicked this off," said Johnson nearly three years

HCA was in good hands after Dr. Thomas Frist Jr. retired from active duty. In 2002 Richard Bracken (left) was promoted to president of HCA, and Jack Bovender (right) became chairman and CEO.

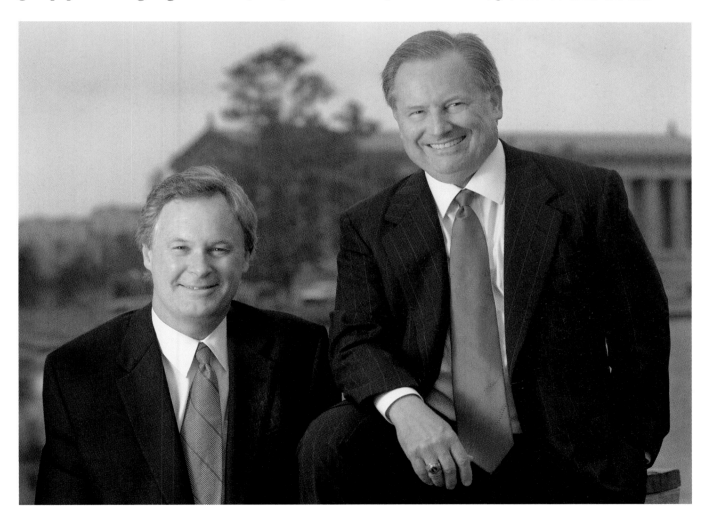

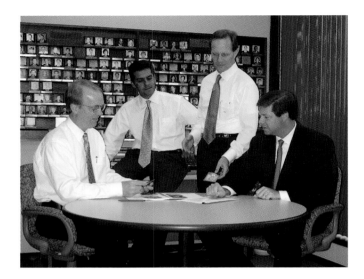

Phil Patton, senior vice president of human resources, Sam Hazen, Western Group president, Jay Grinney, Eastern Group president, and Bruce Moore, senior vice president of operations administration, discuss a hospital CEO candidate. Photos of every hospital CEO hang on the walls of Jack Bovender's and Richard Bracken's offices, a tradition started by Dr. Frist Sr., who frequently noted that hospital administrators (CEOs) are the key to HCA's success.

after the plan was initiated. "We brought in experts from hospitals to help us understand how we should operate in these shared services centers. It was a major risk to the company because it has to do with our revenue stream, our lifeblood. As it's turned out, we've been able to execute the strategy without any major problems. And though it was a high-risk strategy, it's turned out to be very successful."[38]

Patient Safety

At the end of 1999, the Institute of Medicine, a federal agency within the National Institutes of Health, issued a report saying that between 44,000 and 98,000 people a year died because of medical errors in hospitals. The majority of the errors had to do with patients receiving the wrong medication or dosage. Understandably disturbed by these startling numbers, HCA resolved to do everything it could to address these concerns.[39]

Dr. Frank Houser spearheaded HCA's patient safety initiative in the spring of 2000 by bringing in 125 experts from the field, many of them nurses, to offer their feelings and recommendations. HCA's study determined that about 50 percent of the errors were occurring between the time the physician ordered the prescription and the time it reached the pharmacy. Many of these errors occurred because pharmacists couldn't interpret physicians' handwriting; others happened because the doctor made a mistake in the dosage or drug. Another 40 percent of the errors occurred between the time the medication left the pharmacist and the time the nurse administered it. The remaining 10 percent occurred in the pharmacy.

"We came up with two solutions to fix these problems," said Dr. Houser, "both of which had to do with technology."[40]

First, HCA began barcoding the medication so it could be cross-referenced with patients' charts. "Using a wireless rolling laptop and barcode scanner, nurses scan the barcode on the patient's armband and then the barcode on the medication," Dr. Houser explained. "The laptop will tell the nurse whether it's the right dosage for the person's weight and if it's the right time to administer it. The computer also checks the medication against allergies and other drug interactions."[41]

By the spring of 2003, the barcoding system, which used Meditech software, was up and running in 12 hospitals, and HCA hoped to have it running in 65 hospitals by the end of the year.

"It's been very positively received," Dr. Houser said. "It takes some of the burden off the nurses because they know these errors occur, and this gives them a way to double-check the medication they're giving."[42]

HCA's second solution involved physicians using computers to enter prescriptions rather than writing them by hand on prescription pads. "We built the system with a committee of doctors in Meditech, and it took us almost two years to build the software and get all the reviews," said Houser. In the spring of 2003, the new system was being tested in a hospital in Richmond.[43]

An Orderly Transition

After refocusing and restructuring the company he had helped found, on January 8, 2001, Dr. Frist Jr. passed the leadership reins to Jack Bovender, who moved from president and chief operating officer to president and CEO. Bovender became chairman and CEO the following January. Frist Jr. remained on the board of directors, and Richard Bracken became president in addition to his recently appointed duties as chief operating officer. Moving to president of the Western Group was Samuel Hazen, formerly CFO of the group. Jay Grinney remained president of the Eastern Group.

Jack Bovender had the utmost respect for the man he was succeeding. "Tommy is a person of absolute unquestioned integrity," he said. "He is very loyal, and he's a generous person, too, as witnessed by all of his philanthropic activities."[44]

Though Frist Jr. was phasing out his day-to-day duties, he planned to remain involved in the company, helping Bovender and Bracken in any way he could. "This is a huge company," he told a Nashville business publication. "Supporting Jack and Richard is not unlike what my father did up into his eighties, keeping that corporate culture alive and reminding people of your values and beliefs. You're delivering a precious product. These are human lives, and you're caring for people in their weakest moments."[45]

"The key to us going forward is to hang on to the benefits from the Columbia years—the fine people and the incredible assets that came together—and edit out the difficulties," said Bracken. "And that's what we've done over the past several years. We've used those lessons to make us stronger."[46]

Stronger *and* wiser. Bovender spoke of how important it was for HCA to realize and benefit from its shared culture—the common vision of caring, compassion, and quality care. "We worked awfully hard over the last three and a half years to pull this company together," he said. "And now there's a spirit here of people wanting to help each other: a team spirit—because we came through this together."[47]

Health Midwest

On April 1, 2003, HCA acquired 12 hospitals from Health Midwest, a not-for-profit network in Kansas City. Priced at $1.125 billion, it was the largest not-for-profit hospital system ever sold.[48]

Richard Bracken explained what made Health Midwest so appealing to HCA. "We want to have concentrations of hospitals in large cities where we can gain synergies in how they operate and how they position themselves," he said. "We want to be the number one provider in a community or have a chance at being number one with the proper investment and management. With the aging of the baby boomers, we want to make a long-term commitment to an area. Health Midwest was a big system that met those criteria. Also, the system has a good reputation in its community."[49]

"The Health Midwest acquisition was a perfect fit for HCA's strategy," said Western Group President Sam Hazen. "It was the major player in an urban setting. We could acquire this system and, overnight, be the leader in Kansas City. Applying management focus, a solid capital plan, and HCA's systems will turn this into a group of premier hospitals."[50]

Health Midwest had 34 percent market share in a 1.7-million-person market, "which fits beautifully with our strategy to operate complex, tertiary hospitals in large urban areas that have significant population growth," added Bovender.[51]

As so many hospitals had done in the past, Health Midwest chose to be acquired by HCA because it was having financial problems. "The system wasn't generating enough cash flow to keep its facilities modern and up-to-date," said Bovender, adding that HCA would be investing $450 million to upgrade Health Midwest's facilities and provide new equipment. He also noted that the hospitals would now pay taxes, which was a huge benefit to the communities.[52]

Also, because Health Midwest was a not-for-profit, or charity, asset, it compensated the residents of Kansas (where three of the hospitals resided) and Missouri (where 10 hospitals were). Proceeds from the transaction went back into the Kansas City community in the form of two new foundations. Because the hospitals were in both Missouri and Kansas, the $519.5 million in total funds was divided, with $415 million going to Missouri and $104 million going to Kansas.[53]

HCA placed the management of the 12 hospitals of Health Midwest into a newly created Kansas City–based Midwest Division.

DISTINCT AND DISTINGUISHED: THE HCA BOARD OF DIRECTORS

WHEN DONALD MACNAUGHTON CAME TO HCA IN 1977 AS CHAIRMAN AND CEO, HE made it his mission to establish a world-class board of directors. By the time HCA went private in 1989 with its leveraged buyout, the company had one of the best boards in the country, made up of men and women from varied backgrounds whose different perspectives and experiences enhanced the company's management.

In 1997, when HCA began its renaissance, Dr. Frist Jr. added to a strong but small board by recruiting some of the best and brightest business minds in the country.

In 2003 HCA's board of directors comprised 13 outstanding individuals. Four former board members who retired between 1999 and 2003 are also recognized for their leadership during the HCA renaissance.

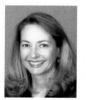
Magdalena H. Averhoff, M.D.
Practicing Physician

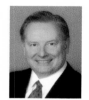
Jack O. Bovender Jr.
Chairman and CEO, HCA

Richard M. Bracken
President and COO, HCA

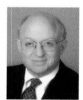
Martin Feldstein
Professor of Economics, Harvard University; President and CEO, National Bureau of Economic Research

Thomas F. Frist Jr., M.D.
Cofounder, HCA

Frederick W. Gluck
Senior Counselor, McKinsey & Company, Inc.; Retired Vice Chairman, Bechtel Group, Inc.; Retired Managing Director, McKinsey & Company

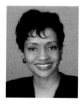
Glenda A. Hatchett
Host of Syndicated Television Court Show; Retired Chief Judge, Fulton County Juvenile Court

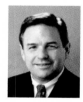
Charles O. Holliday Jr.
Chairman and CEO, DuPont

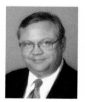
T. Michael Long
Partner, Brown Brothers Harriman & Company

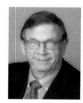
John H. McArthur
Retired Dean of Harvard University Graduate School of Business

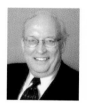
Kent C. Nelson
Retired Chairman and CEO, United Parcel Service

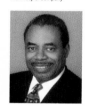
Frank S. Royal, M.D.
Practicing Physician

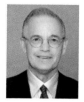
Harold T. Shapiro
President Emeritus, Princeton University

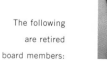
The following are retired board members:

Elaine L. Chao
Distinguished Fellow, The Heritage Foundation

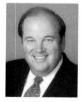
J. Michael Cook
Retired Chairman and CEO, Deloitte & Touche LLP

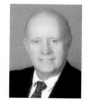
Thomas S. Murphy
Retired Chairman and CEO, Capital Cities/ABC, Inc.

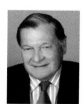
Carl E. Reichardt
Vice Chairman of Ford Motor Company; Retired Chairman and CEO, Wells Fargo & Company.

Back to the Future

As early as 1999, business writers were speaking of a transformation of HCA's character and culture, but perhaps the recent years of the company are better understood as repossession and renewal. The world of healthcare had changed dramatically in the 35 years after HCA's founding, and HCA played a great part. As the largest investor-owned hospital company in the world during that period, it presented a strong example of the prospects and capabilities of the free market and reinforced the importance of timeless and essential principles: receiving patients with compassion and kindness.[54]

Jack Massey had put people first during the Great Depression when he extended credit to doctors while he himself was asking for patience from those to whom he owed money. Dr. Thomas Frist Sr. based his great company on compassion for patients in hospitals. The third of the founders, Dr. Thomas Frist Jr., kept in view these principles of trust in people to do the right thing and the wish and will of healthcare providers to extend to patients the loving as well as the learned touch. Jack Bovender and Richard Bracken continued the traditions set down by the founders and combined the lessons learned from their mentors with lessons learned from HCA's successes and tribulations.

"We are firm in what we believe in," said Bracken in the spring of 2003. "We know what works and what doesn't work."[55]

Though Bracken observed that HCA was "better now than we've ever been," he also acknowledged that all of the strategies and initiatives HCA had been implementing in the past five years were ongoing. "These agendas are never over," he said. "I don't think we'll ever be a company that takes its eye off what we're all about. We're always going to be focused on service, patients, physicians, running the best hospitals. And we'll always be looking at how to improve those agendas."[56]

Or, as Bovender said, "Our primary concern is making sure that the patient and the patient's family are well cared for. That was true 35 years ago, and it's true today. All the other stuff is noise."[57]

A TIME LINE OF KEY EVENTS

1961: Dr Thomas Frist Sr. opens Park View Hospital in Nashville.

1978: Donald MacNaughton becomes chairman and chief executive officer. By the end of its 10th year, HCA operates more than 120 facilities in 25 states and four foreign countries. It holds management contracts with 30 hospitals.

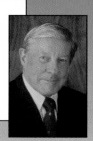

1992: HCA goes public again.

1965: Lyndon B. Johnson signs the Medicare bill that provides hospital and medical insurance for Americans over the age of 65, regardless of their economic means.

1973: After only five years in business, HCA has 57 hospitals in operation in 13 states.

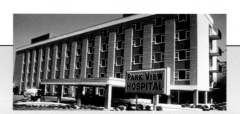

1987: HCA spins off 104 hospitals to an employee stock ownership plan to form Nashville-based HealthTrust, with Clayton McWhorter at the helm.

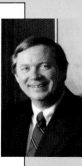

1961

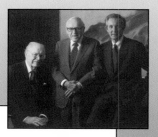

1968: Dr. Thomas Frist Sr., his son Dr. Thomas Frist Jr., and Jack Massey found Hospital Corporation of America in Nashville.

1970: John Hill becomes president of HCA.

1983: Congress passes Medicare amendments. Under the law's prospective payment system, hospitals will be reimbursed only a predetermined amount for treating a diagnosed illness (DRG).

1989: Frist Jr. takes HCA private, leading a $5.1 billion leveraged buyout. As a private company, HCA rebuilds its strength.

IN THE EVOLUTION OF HCA

1994: Columbia and HCA merge to form Columbia/HCA. Richard Scott becomes president and CEO of the new entity.

1998: The company launches its Ethics and Compliance program.

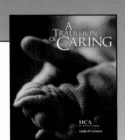

2000: The company reaches initial agreements with the U.S. Justice Department to settle all criminal and several civil allegations.

2001: Frist Jr. retires. Jack Bovender moves from president and CEO to chairman and CEO. Richard Bracken becomes president and chief operating officer.

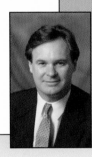

1998–1999: The company begins restructuring, culminating with the spin-offs of LifePoint and Triad in May 1999. HCA is right-sized to 180 hospitals, and operating results return to mid-teen levels by 1999.

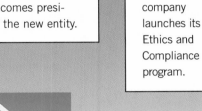

1995: Columbia/HCA grows rapidly, with HealthTrust rejoining the network. By the end of the year, its network includes more than 340 hospitals, 135 surgery centers, and 550 home healthcare locations.

2003

2002: The company settles all remaining issues with the Justice Department. HCA earnings are up 30 percent, the fourth consecutive year of mid-teens-plus growth. HCA's stock price reaches an all-time high.

March 1997: The federal government begins investigating Columbia/HCA's business practices, starting in El Paso.

2003: HCA acquires Health Midwest, a 12-hospital network based in Kansas City. By now, HCA's initiatives to strengthen the company are in place, and its operations, comprising 190 hospitals, are stronger than ever.

July 1997: Frist Jr. comes out of retirement and returns to his role as chairman and CEO. Jack Bovender rejoins the company as president and COO. The new leaders focus on core assets and divest noncore assets and hospitals. They unveil the new mission and values statement that renews the standard of putting the patient first. They also initiate a $5 billion share repurchase plan.

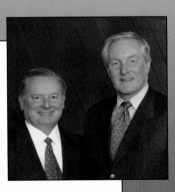

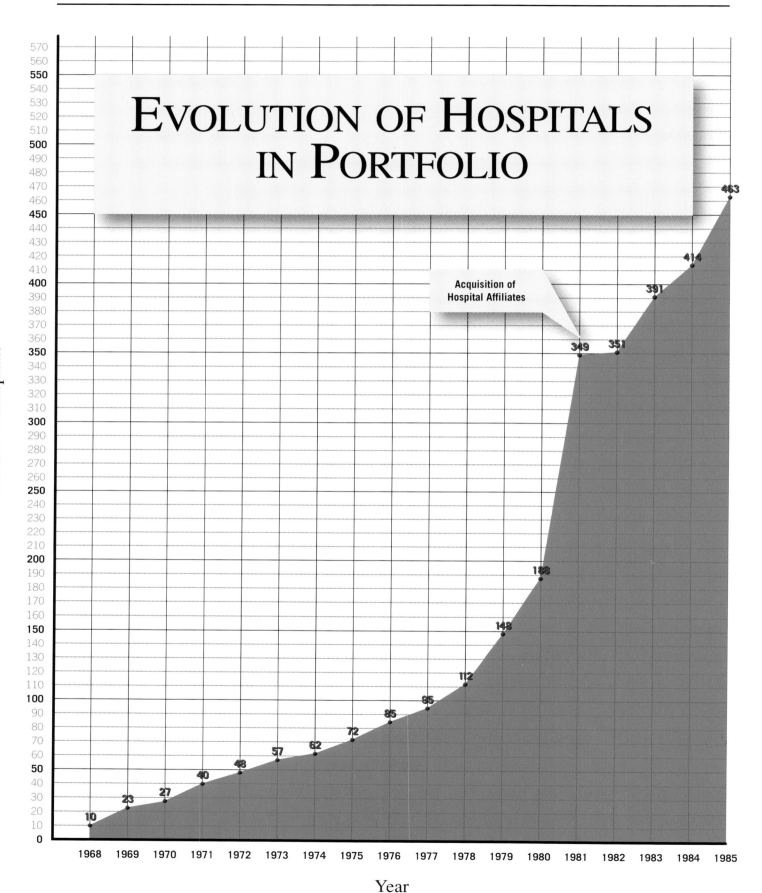

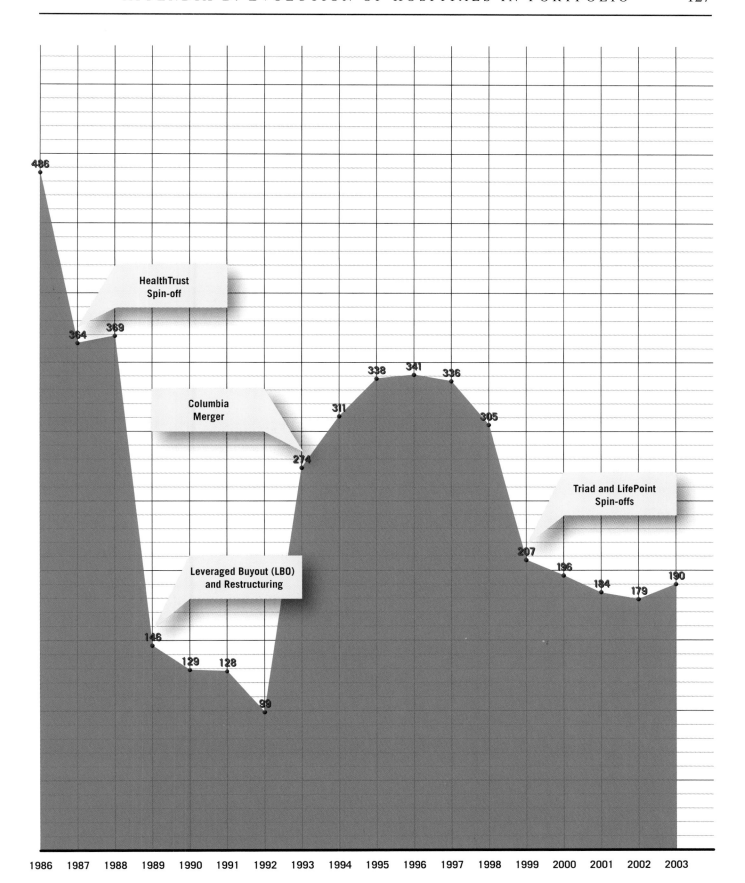

486

HealthTrust
Spin-off

364   369

Columbia
Merger

338   341   336

311

305

274

Triad and LifePoint
Spin-offs

207
196

Leveraged Buyout (LBO)
and Restructuring

146

129   128

184
179   190

99

1986 1987 1988 1989 1990 1991 1992 1993 1994 1995 1996 1997 1998 1999 2000 2001 2002 2003

Year (continued)

DIRECTORS OF HCA

Name and title (as of last year on HCA board)	Years served
George G. Alexander, M.D., physician	1968–1978
Max M. Diamond, M.D., physician	1968–1984
William R. Fowler, M.D., physician	1968–1971
Thomas F. Frist Sr., M.D., HCA founder, vice chairman, and chief medical officer	1968–1983
Thomas F. Frist Jr., M.D., HCA founder, retired chairman, president, and CEO	1968–current
Richard Harrell, businessman	1968–1970
Thomas N. P. Johns, M.D., physician	1968–1985
Jack C. Massey, HCA founder and chairman	1968–1981
Robert E. McClellan, M.D., physician	1968–1969
C. George Mercy, HCA senior vice president	1968–1979
Cleo M. Miller, M. D., physician	1968–1970
John C. Neff, HCA president and CEO	1968–1975
William L. Taylor, M.D., physician	1968–1971
David G. Williamson Jr., HCA vice chairman	1968–1985
Millard Bartels, counsel, Alcorn, Bakewell & Smith	1970–1982
John A. Hill, former HCA president and CEO	1970–1982
Richard S. Perkins, chairman, Skandinaviska Enskilda Banken International Corp.	1970–1983
Robert Anderson, chairman and CEO, Rockwell International Corp.	1971–1988
Robert P. Brueck, retired HCA executive vice president; president, Center for Health Studies	1971–1979
Ira H. Degenhardt, M.D., physician	1971
Hugh H. Hanson, M.D., physician	1971–1972
J. Francis Morgan, businessman	1971–1973
Leo H. Strauss, businessman	1971
Carl E. Reichardt, retired chairman and CEO of Wells Fargo; vice chairman of Ford Motor	1972–2003
Winfield Dunn, HCA senior vice president	1974–1984
Nancy Dickerson, television journalist, author, and lecturer	1976–1977

Robert Q. Marston, president, University of Florida 1976–1977
William C. Weaver Jr., retired chairman and CEO, NLT Corp. 1977–1978
John D. deButts, retired chairman and CEO, AT&T 1978–1985
Donald S. MacNaughton, retired HCA chairman and CEO .1978–1986
       former HealthTrust chairman of the executive committee . . .1994–1997
Charles J. Kane, retired chairman, Third National Corp. 1979–1995
Frank Borman, chairman and CEO, Patlex Corp.; former astronaut. 1980–1988
Owen B. Butler, chairman, Procter & Gamble Co. 1980–1988
Barbara M. Clark, The Massey Companies 1981–1988
Irving S. Shapiro, partner, Skadden, Arps, Slate, Meagher & Flom 1981–1988
Frank T. Cary, retired chairman and CEO, IBM Corp. 1982–1988
Frank S. Royal, M.D., physician 1982–current
R. Clayton McWhorter, HCA president and CEO 1983–1986
     chairman, HCA; chairman and CEO, Clayton Associates 1994–1999
Donald V. Seibert, retired chairman and CEO, J. C. Penney Co. 1985–1988
Joe B. Wyatt, chancellor, Vanderbilt University 1985–1988
Martin Feldstein, professor of economics, Harvard University 1986–1988
Clifton C. Garvin Jr., retired chairman and CEO, Exxon Corp. 1986–1988
Charles N. Martin Jr., HCA executive vice president 1986
John L. Thornton, M.D., physician 1986–1988
Roger E. Mick, HCA senior vice president and CFO 1987–1991
Charles T. Harris III, general partner, The Goldman Sachs Group 1989–1993
Richard E. Rainwater, independent investor 1989–1992
T. Michael Long, partner, Brown Brothers Harriman & Co. .1991–current
Jack O. Bovender Jr., HCA executive vice president and chief operating officer 1992–1995
       HCA chairman and CEO 1999–current
Richard L. Scott, Columbia/HCA chairman and CEO 1993–1996
Magdalena H. Averhoff, M.D., physician 1993–current
J. David Grissom, chairman, Mayfair Capital 1993–1994
Ethan Jackson, investor 1993
John W. Landrum, owner, Springlake Farms 1993–1995
Darla D. Moore, investor 1993–1994
Rodman W. Moorhead III, senior managing director, E. M. Warburg Pincus & Co. 1993–1995
Carl F. Pollard, Columbia/HCA chairman of the executive committee 1993–1994
Robert D. Walter, chairman and CEO, Cardinal Health 1993–1995
William T. Young, chairman, W. T. Young 1993–1997
Richard W. Hanselman, retired chairman, president, and CEO, Genesco 1994
Sister Judith Ann Karam, Sisters of Charity of St. Augustine 1995–1997
Frederick W. Gluck, senior counselor, McKinsey & Co. 1997–current
John H. McArthur, retired dean of Harvard University Graduate School of Business . . .1997–current
Kent C. Nelson, retired chairman and CEO, United Parcel Service 1997–current
Martin Feldstein, professor of economics, Harvard University 1998–current
Thomas S. Murphy, chairman and CEO emeritus, Capital Cities/ABC 1998–2001
Elaine L. Chao, distinguished fellow, The Heritage Foundation 1999
J. Michael Cook, retired chairman and CEO, DeLoitte & Touche 1999–2003
Glenda A. Hatchett, former chief judge, Fulton County Juvenile Court 1999–current
Harold T. Shapiro, president emeritus, Princeton University .2000–current
Charles O. Holliday Jr., chairman and CEO, DuPont 2002–current
Richard M. Bracken, HCA president and chief operating officer 2003–current

NOTES TO SOURCES

Chapter One

1. Information provided by Dr. Thomas F. Frist Jr., June 2003.
2. Ibid.
3. *Nashville Banner,* 5 November 1990.
4. Ida Cooney, *Hospital Corporation of America: A History,* unpublished manuscript.
5. *Nashville Banner,* 9 July 1981.
6. Cooney, *Hospital Corporation of America.*
7. *Nashville Tennessean,* 5 January 1998.
8. Samuel S. Riven, M.D., *Worthy Lives: Medical Men and Women at Vanderbilt in the 1930s* (Nashville: Vanderbilt University Medical Center, 1993), 31.
9. Cooney, *Hospital Corporation of America.*
10. Ibid.
11. Dr. Thomas Frist Sr., interview by Deborah Cooney, transcript, 6 June 1968, 22 June 1968, and 25 July 1978, Hospital Corporation of America.
12. Cooney, *Hospital Corporation of America.*
13. *Nashville Tennessean,* 5 January 1998.
14. Frist Sr., interview, 6 June 1968, 22 June 1968, and 25 July 1978.
15. Ibid.
16. *Nashville Tennessean,* 18 December 1961; Bill Carey, *Fortunes, Fiddles, and Fried Chicken* (Franklin, Tennessee: Hillsboro Press, 2000), 351.
17. Dr. Thomas Frist Sr., HCA History (videotape) no date; *Nashville Banner,* 18 December 1961; *Nashville Banner,* 9 July 1981.
18. *Nashville Tennessean,* 18 December 1961.
19. Cooney, *Hospital Corporation of America.*
20. *Nashville Tennessean,* 15 August 1967.
21. Frist Sr., interview, 6 June 1968, 22 June 1968, and 25 July 1978.
22. *Nashville Tennessean,* 15 August 1967; *Nashville Tennessean,* 5 January 1998.
23. Cooney, *Hospital Corporation of America.*
24. Frist Sr., interview, 6 June 1968, 22 June 1968, and 25 July 1978.
25. Carey, *Fortunes, Fiddles, and Fried Chicken,* 234–47.
26. *Nashville Tennessean,* 19 February 1990.
27. Information provided by Frist Jr., June 2003.
28. Ibid.
29. Ibid.
30. Cooney, *Hospital Corporation of America.*
31. Dr. Thomas F. Frist Jr., interview by Deborah Cooney, transcript, 22 May 1978 and 17 June 1978, Hospital Corporation of America.
32. Cooney, *Hospital Corporation of America.*
33. Ibid.
34. Ibid.
35. Carey, *Fortunes, Fiddles, and Fried Chicken,* 352; Certificate of Incorporation, Hospital Corporation of America, Department of State, State of Tennessee, 1 May 1968.
36. Jack C. Massey, interview by Deborah Cooney, transcript, 22 July 1978, Hospital Corporation of America.
37. *Nashville Tennessean,* 25 June 1968.

38. Frist Jr., interview, 22 May 1978 and 17 June 1978.
39. David G. Williamson Jr., interview by Deborah Cooney, transcript, 26 April 1978 and 8 May 1978, Hospital Corporation of America.
40. Ibid.
41. Cathy Schulze, "Williamson Brings Enthusiasm, Expertise to HCA Career," *Nashville Banner*, 10 October 1985.
42. Frist Jr., interview, 22 May 1978 and 17 June 1978.
43. *Nashville Banner*, 18 October 1968.
44. Frist Jr., interview, 22 May 1978 and 17 June 1978.
45. Frist Sr., interview, 6 June 1968, 22 June 1968, and 25 July 1978.
46. Cooney, *Hospital Corporation of America*; Robert P. Brueck, interview by Deborah Cooney, transcript, 2 May 1978 and 10 May 1978, Hospital Corporation of America.
47. Frist Jr., interview, 22 May 1978 and 17 June 1978.
48. Ibid.
49. James G. Leonard, interview by Deborah Cooney, transcript, 20 March 1978, Hospital Corporation of America.
50. *Nashville Banner*, 4 March 1988.
51. Frist Jr., interview, 22 May 1978 and 17 June 1978.
52. *Nashville Banner*, 4 March 1988.

Chapter Two

1. Donald W. Fish, interview by Deborah Cooney, transcript, 20 March 1978 and 27 July 1978, Hospital Corporation of America.
2. Frist Sr., interview, 6 June 1968, 22 June 1968, and 25 July 1978.
3. *Nashville Banner*, 12 April 1994; *New York Times*, 14 April 1994; Frist Jr. interview, 22 May 1978 and 17 June 1978.
4. Dr. Thomas F. Frist Jr., interview by the author, recording, 12 March 2001.
5. Secretary of State, Tennessee Blue Book, 1979–1980 (Nashville: Secretary of State, n.d.).
6. Sam A. Brooks Jr., interview by Deborah Cooney, transcript, 6 May 1978 and 23 May 1978, Hospital Corporation of America.
7. Fish, interview.
8. Ibid.
9. Brooks, interview.
10. John C. Neff, interview by Deborah Cooney, transcript, 24 April 1978, Hospital Corporation of America.
11. Ibid.
12. Ibid.
13. Carey, *Fortunes, Fiddles, and Fried Chicken*, 356–57.
14. "Southern Fried Hospitals," *Forbes*, 15 November 1976, 113.
15. John A. Hill, interview by Deborah Cooney, transcript, 13 April 1978, Hospital Corporation of America.
16. Brueck, interview.
17. *Nashville Tennessean*, 25 June 1968; *Nashville Tennessean*, 13 November 1968; HCA 1973 Annual Report, 16.
18. "A Profit Boost for Hospitals," *Business Week*, 2 October 1971; "Rx: $$$$$," *Forbes*, 1 May 1973, 51.
19. Ibid.
20. "Hospital Corp. of America Slated for Healthy Advance," *Barron's*, 24 February 1975, 40.
21. "Hospitals That Heal Themselves," *Newsweek*, 28 May 1973, 72; "Hospital Corp. of America Slated," 40.
22. Charles E. Rosenberg, *The Care of Strangers; The Rise of America's Hospital System* (New York: Basic Books, 1987), 327–32.
23. "Free-Enterprise Answer?" *Forbes*, 15 January 1976, 4.
24. Brueck, interview.
25. Rosemary Stevens, *In Sickness and in Wealth* (New York: Basic Books, 1989), 232–36; Charles Hurd, *The Compact History of the American Red Cross* (New York: Hawthorn Books, 1959), 290.
26. HCA 1972 Annual Report, 10.
27. Frist Jr., interview, 22 May 1978 and 17 June 1978.
28. James D. Snyder, "Hospital Chains: Up, Around, and Eating Well," *Sales Management*, 20 August 1973, 24.
29. Sandy Lutz and E. Preston Gee, *Columbia/HCA: Healthcare on Overdrive* (New York: McGraw Hill, 1998), 15; "Food Man Whips up a Chain of Hospitals," *Business Week*, 30 May 1970, 44; "Making Hospitals Pay," *Forbes*, 15 October 1970, 76–77.
30. HCA 1971 Annual Report, 19.
31. Brooks, interview.
32. HCA 1969 Annual Report, unpaginated; HCA 1971 Annual Report, 27.
33. Milton Johnson, interview by the author, recording, 9 February 2001, Write Stuff Enterprises.
34. HCA 1971 Annual Report 23.
35. HCA 1972 Annual Report, 23, 27; "Hospital Corp. of America Slated," 40.
36. Johnson, interview, 9 February 2001.
37. Brueck, interview.
38. Frist Sr., interview, 6 June 1968, 22 June 1968, and 25 July 1978.

39. Hill, interview.
40. Williamson Jr., interview.
41. HCA 1972 Annual Report, 5; HCA 1973 Annual Report, 18, 25.
42. Brueck, interview.
43. Ibid.
44. HCA 1973 Annual Report, 7.
45. *Wall Street Journal*, 19 March 1972.
46. C. George Mercy, interview by Deborah Cooney, transcript, 19 April 1978, Hospital Corporation of America.
47. Robert C. Crosby, interview by Deborah Cooney, transcript, 17 May 1978 and 25 July 1978, Hospital Corporation of America.
48. Ibid.
49. Hill, interview.
50. Mercy, interview.
51. Frist Jr. interview, 22 May 1978 and 17 June 1978.
52. HCA 1974 Annual Report, 17–18.
53. Crosby, interview.
54. HCA 1971 Annual Report, 13; *New York Times*, 6 October 1971.
55. Mercy, interview.
56. Brueck, interview.
57. HCA 1973 Annual Report, 26.
58. Ibid, 7–8; HCA Annual Report 1971, 24.

Chapter Two Sidebar:
Physician Relations

1. HCA 1972 Annual Report, 22–23.
2. HCA 1971 Annual Report, 19–20.
3. Information provided by Victor Campbell to Melody Maysonet, 7 December 2001.
4. HCA 1972 Annual Report, 16–19; HCA 1973 Annual Report, 17.
5. Mercy, interview.

Chapter Two Sidebar:
Government Enters Healthcare

1. Paul F. Starr, *The Social Transformation of American Medicine* (New York: Basic Books, 1982), 375; Eric Foner and Jon A. Garraty, eds., "Medicare," *The Reader's Companion to American History* (Boston: Houghton-Mifflin, 1991), 716–718.

Chapter Three

1. Frist Jr., interview, 12 March 2001.
2. Carl George, interview by the author, recording, 9 February 2001, Write Stuff Enterprises.
3. Helen King Cummings, interview by Melody Maysonet, recording, 13 May 2002, Write Stuff Enterprises.
4. "Post Meeting Report, Annual Meeting of the Shareholders," HCA, 18 April 1980, 14.
5. Victor Campbell, interview by the author, recording, 12 March 2001, Write Stuff Enterprises.
6. George, interview.
7. Jim Fitzgerald, interview by the author, recording, 9 February 2001, Write Stuff Enterprises.
8. Jack Bovender, interview by the author, recording, 8 February 2001, Write Stuff Enterprises.
9. Victor Campbell, interview, 12 March 2001.
10. Cummings, interview.
11. Noel Williams, interview by Richard F. Hubbard, recording, 10 August 2001, Write Stuff Enterprises.
12. Richard Bracken, interview by Melody Maysonet, recording, 19 March 2003, Write Stuff Enterprises.

13. R. Clayton McWhorter, interview by Marc K. Stengel, transcript, 1 July 1986, Hospital Corporation of America.
14. Steve Riven, speech to present the Vanderbilt Alumnist Award to Thomas Frist Jr., n.d.
15. HCA 1969 Annual Report, unpaginated.
16. HCA 1974 Annual Report, 5–6.
17. "Quality Assurance Department" in Hospital Corporation of America, Interim Report, Three Months Ended March 31, 1975, unpaginated.
18. HCA 1969 Annual Report, unpaginated; HCA 1978 Annual Report, 21.
19. Frist Jr., interview, 22 May 1978 and 17 June 1978.
20. HCA 1974 Annual Report, 32; HCA 1976 Annual Report, 2; HCA 1977 Annual Report, 2; Paul B. Brown, "Band Aids by the Box Car," *Forbes*, 31 August 1981, 89.
21. HCA 1976 Annual Report, 14, 15; HCA 1977 Annual Report, 5; HCA 1978 Annual Report, 8; James Summerville, *Educating Black Doctors; A History of Meharry Medical College* (Tuscaloosa: University of Alabama Press, 1983).
22. "The Money in Curing Hospitals," *Business Week*, 25 June 1979, 58.
23. *Wall Street Journal*, 12 May 1976; *Wall Street Journal*, 22 April 1977; HCA 1977 Annual Report, 2–3.
24. R. Clayton McWhorter, interview by Deborah Cooney, transcript, 25 May 1978 and 5 July 1978, Hospital Corporation of America.
25. Ibid.

26. Ibid.
27. Post Meeting Report on the Tenth Anniversary Annual Meeting of Stockholders, 21 April, 1978, Hospital Corporation of America
28. John Hindelong, interview by Melody Maysonet, recording, 21 December 2001, Write Stuff Enterprises.
29. Campbell to Maysonet, 7 December 2001.
30. Post Meeting Report, 21 April 1978.
31. Ibid.
32. HCA 1978 Annual Report, 6; *Wall Street Journal*, 29 June 1978; *New York Times*, 29 June 1978.
33. Donald S. MacNaughton, interview by Marc K. Stengel, transcript, 7 May 1986, Hospital Corporation of America.
34. Dr. Thomas F. Frist Jr., interview by Marc K. Stengel, transcript, 2 April 1986, Hospital Corporation of America.
35. MacNaughton, interview.
36. Frist Jr., interview, 2 April 1986.
37. Frist Sr., interview, 6 June 1968, 22 June 1968, and 25 July 1978.
38. Frist Jr., interview, 12 March 2001; Frist Jr., interview, 2 April 1986.
39. McWhorter, interview, 1 July 1986, HCA.
40. Post Meeting Report, 21 April 1978.

Chapter Four

1. Frist Jr., interview, 2 April 1986.
2. Cummings, interview.
3. Frist Jr., interview, 2 April 1986.
4. Ibid.
5. Dr. Thomas F. Frist Jr., interview by the author, recording, 8 February 2001, Write Stuff Enterprises.

6. Carey, *Fortunes, Fiddles & Fried Chicken*, 359, 360.
7. McWhorter, interview, 1 July 1986.
8. Frist Jr., interview, 12 March 2001.
9. HCA 1982 Annual Report.
10. HCA 1982 Annual Report, 3–10; HCA 1982 First Quarter Report, 8–11; HCA 1983 Annual Report, 4, 6; HCA 1984 Annual Report, unpaginated; "Hospital Corp. Operates on Its Debt," *Business Week*, 29 March 1982, 150; "Margins for Health," *Financial World*, April 1984, 30.
11. HCA 1983 Annual Report; HCA 1984 Annual Report.
12. HCA 1985 Annual Report.
13. HCA 1984 Annual Report.
14. Ibid.
15. Ibid.
16. HCA 1983 Annual Report, 10, 12; HCA 1984 Annual Report; HCA 1985 Annual Report, 4; *Nashville Banner*, 15 February 1985.
17. HCA 1984 Annual Report.
18. HCA 1983 Annual Report, 8, 10.
19. HCA 1982 Annual Report, 7; HCA 1984 Annual Report; HCA 1985 Annual Report, 15; HCA 1986 Annual Report, 3; Michael McFadden, "Health Purveyors That Look Hale," *Fortune*, 26 May 1986, 147; Jennifer Bingham Hill, "Hospital Corp. to Reduce Beverly Enterprises Stake," *Wall Street Journal*, 24 May 1985.
20. HCA 1986 Annual Report, 7.
21. Ibid., 14.
22. Ibid., 10; HCA 1984 Annual Report; HCA 1985 Annual Report, 8; *Nashville Tennessean*, 8 November 1984.
23. HCA 1984 Annual Report; *Nashville Tennessean*, 3

January 1985; *Nashville Tennessean*, 1 August 1985; *Nashville Banner*, 1 August 1985.
24. *Wall Street Journal*, 1 April 1985; *Tennessean*, 1 April 1985; *Nashville Banner*, 1 April 1985; David Barkholz, "Backlash Could Cost American Millions," *Modern Healthcare*, 26 April 1985, 22; Ford S. Worthy, "A Merger That Pains Hospitals," *Fortune*, 24 June 1985, 106–197; David Barkholz, "American Sales Could Drop $500 Million in Backlash to Proposed HCA Merger," *Modern Healthcare*, 19 July 1985, 22–23.
25. Mark Tatge, "PPS Stalled HCA-American Talks," *Modern Healthcare*, 26 April 1985, 22.
26. *Nashville Banner*, 13 June 1985; *Wall Street Journal*, 16 July 1985; Ellen E. Spragins and Rebecca Aikman, "A Shattered Dream at American Hospital Supply," *Business Week*, 29 July 1985, 27–28.
27. Victor Campbell, interview by Marc K. Stengel, transcript, 11 February 1986, Hospital Corporation of America.
28. Campbell, interview, 12 March 2001.
29. Ibid.
30. MacNaughton, interview.
31. HCA 1986 Annual Report, 3–4; HCA 1987 Annual Report, 2, 11; *New York Times*, 5 March 1986; *Wall Street Journal*, 5 March 1986.

Chapter Four Sidebar: Foundations for Giving

1. Peter Bird, interview by Melody Maysonet, recording, 3 May 2002, Write Stuff Enterprises.

2. Ibid.
3. Ibid.
4. "The HCA Foundation,"
   Hcacaring.org, June 2002.
5. *Caring for the Community*,
   2000 Community
   Contribution Report, HCA
   Foundation.

Chapter Five

1. HCA 1983 Annual Report, 3;
   HCA 1984 Annual Report;
   Nashville Banner, 15
   February 1985; *Wall Street
   Journal*, 10 October 1985.
2. Campbell, interview, 12 March
   2001.
3. HCA 1985 Annual Report, 2;
   "Notice of Special Meeting of
   Shareholders to Be Held on
   March 15, 1989," HCA, 129.
4. Cummings, interview.
5. Trish Lindler, interview by the
   author, recording, 9 February
   2001, Write Stuff Enterprises.
6. Information provided by Victor
   Campbell to Melody
   Maysonet, 14 March 2003.
7. *New York Times*, 8 October
   1985; *New York Times*, 24
   October 1985; Mark Rust,
   "For-Profit Hospital Stocks
   Take Wall Street Beating,"
   American Medical News, 18
   October 1985, 2; *Los Angeles
   Times*, 16 November 1985;
   Wall Street Journal, 3
   September 1985; *Wall Street
   Journal*, 3 October 1985; *Wall
   Street Journal*, 18 November
   1985; Teri Shahoda,
   "Theories Abound on HCA's
   Future," *Hospitals*, 1
   November 1985, 21–23.
8. McWhorter, interview, 1 July
   1986.
9. Ibid.
10. Thomas Frist Sr., interview by
    Marc K. Stengel, transcript, 6
    May 1986, Hospital
    Corporation of America.

11. Information provided by
    Victor Campbell to Melody
    Maysonet, April 2002; "HCA
    Announces Financing
    Commitments and Board
    Approval for Repositioning
    Plan," HCA investor report,
    31 May 1987.
12. Campbell to Maysonet, April
    2002.
13. HCA 1987 Annual Report, 2.
14. Ibid, 11.
15. Michael Abramowitz,
    "Prognosis Is Uncertain for
    Employee Ownership of 104
    HCA Hospitals," *Washington
    Post*, 28 June 1987.
16. "HCA Sells 104 Hospitals to
    Employee-Owned Company,"
    U.P.I., 17 September 1987.
17. Abramowitz, "Prognosis is
    Uncertain."
18. Christopher Palmeri, "Every
    Dog Has His Day," *Forbes*, 28
    March 1994.
19. Steve Rogers, "Spreading the
    Gospel of HealthTrust,"
    Advantage, July 1990.
20. Carey, *Fortunes, Fiddles &
    Fried Chicken*, 442.
21. Rogers, "Spreading the Gospel."
22. Palmeri, "Every Dog has His
    Day."
23. "1987 Third Quarter Results
    Reflect Gain on Hospital
    Divestiture," HCA investor
    report, 14 October 1987.
24. "HCA Sells 104 Hospitals."
25. "Closing Expected Later
    Today for HealthTrust
    Acquisition of 104 HCA
    Hospitals for $2.1 billion,"
    HCA investor report, 17
    September 1987.
26. Laura Sachar, "Southern
    Comfort," *Financial World*, 15
    December 1987, 30
27. "HCA Completes Stock
    Repurchase," Associated
    Press, 5 January 1988.
28. Sachar, "Southern Comfort,"
    30; Dean Foust, "Suddenly,

HCA Is Talking LBO," *Business
    Week*, 3 October 1988, 37.
29. Hindelong, interview.
30. Campbell to Maysonet, April
    2002.
31. *New York Times*, 16
    September 1988.
32. Campbell to Maysonet, April
    2002.
33. *New York Times*, 14 October
    1988; Robert Teitelman,
    "Dear Mr. Jones," *Financial
    World*, 31 May 1988, 20; Frist
    Jr., interview, 8 February
    2001.
34. Lutz and Gee, *Columbia/HCA*,
    28
35. Campbell to Maysonet, April
    2002.
36. *New York Times*, 22
    November 1988; Stuart
    Flack, "A Crazy Deal?"
    Forbes, 24 July 1989; Lutz
    and Gee, *Columbia/HCA*, 28.
37. Lutz and Gee, *Columbia/HCA*,
    28; *New York Times*, 22
    November 1988.

Chapter Six

1. Carey, *Fortunes, Fiddles &
   Fried Chicken*, 441.
2. *New York Times*, 23 November
   1998; *Wall Street Journal*, 18
   June 1991.
3. *Wall Street Journal*, 13 June
   1989; *Wall Street Journal*, 4
   October 1989; *Wall Street
   Journal*, 4 February 1991;
   Wall Street Journal, 18 June
   1991; *Wall Street Journal*, 12
   November 1992; Carey,
   *Fortunes, Fiddles & Fried
   Chicken*, 442.
4. Lutz and Gee, *Columbia/HCA*,
   29.
5. Ibid.
6. Ibid, 30.
7. Flack, "A Crazy Deal?", 58;
   "HCA: Another Painful
   Experience, *Financial World*,
   23 January 1990, 18.

8. Lutz and Gee, *Columbia/HCA,*
30–31.
9. Chuck Hawkins, "The Golden
Road from LBO to IPO,"
Business Week, 27 January
1992, 64; HCA 1992 Annual
Report, 5.
10. Hawkins, "The Golden Road,"
64–65.
11. Lauren R. Rublin, "Mending
HCA: Restructuring Plan Puts
Hospital Corp. on Recovery's
Road," *Barron's,* 22 August
1988; HCA 1992 Annual
Report, 11.
12. Bovender, interview, 8
February 2001.
13. Bill Rutherford, interview by
Richard F. Hubbard,
recording, 10 August 2001,
Write Stuff Enterprises.
14. Richard Bracken, interview by
the author, recording, 9
August 2001, Write Stuff
Enterprises.
15. Hawkins, "The Golden Road,"
64.
16. *New York Times,* 4 January
1992; *Wall Street Journal,* 16
January 1992; *Wall Street
Journal,* 21 September 1992;
Hawkins, "The Golden Road,"
64.
17. HCA 1992 Annual Report, 5.
18. *Wall Street Journal,* 16
January 1992; *Wall Street
Journal,* 5 March 1992.
19. HCA 1992 Annual Report, 6.
20. *Wall Street Journal,* 17
November 1992; Bovender,
interview, 8 February 2001.
21. Jack O. Bovender Jr.,
"Viewpoint: A Look at the
Hospital Administrator," *Health
Care Management Review,* 11,
no. 4, 1986, 92, 93–94.

Chapter Seven

1. Lutz and Gee, *Columbia/HCA,*
80-81; Frist Jr., interview, 12
March 2001.

2. Columbia Hospital Corporation
1993 Annual Report, 2.
3. David Anderson, interview by
the author, recording, 9
February 2001, Write Stuff
Enterprises.
4. Ibid.
5. Columbia/HCA 1993 Annual
Report, 12; *Wall Street
Journal,* 12 July 1994.
6. Rosalyn Elton, interview by the
author, recording, 9 February
2001, Write Stuff Enterprises.
7. Wendy Zellner, Mike McNamee,
and David Greising, "And
Now, Monolith Hospital,"
Business Week, no. 3325, 33.
8. Ibid; Lutz and Gee,
Columbia/HCA, 82.
9. "Boy Wonder," 25 October
1993, 242.
10. Frist Jr., interview, 12 March
2001.
11. *New York Times,* 3 October
1993; *New York Times,* 4
October 1993.
12. Ibid.
13. *New York Times,* 4 October
1993.
14. *Wall Street Journal,* 5 October
1993; Lutz and Gee,
Columbia/HCA, 59.
15. Zachary Schiller and Maria
Mallory, "HCA-Columbia: A
Concorde or a Blimp?"
Business Week, 18 October
1993, 36; *Wall Street Journal,*
12 July 1994.

**Chapter Seven Sidebar:
Columbia's Beginnings**

1. Lutz and Gee, *Columbia/HCA,*
69–70.
2. *Wall Street Journal,* 5
October 1993; Schiller
and Mallory, "HCA-
Columbia," 36.
3. Columbia Hospital Corporation
1991 Annual Report, 12.
4. Columbia Hospital Corporation
1990 Annual Report, 1, 25.

5. Lutz and Gee, *Columbia/HCA,*
77, 79, 82.

Chapter Eight

1. Columbia/HCA 1994 Annual
Report, 3.
2. Ibid, 3–4.
3. Columbia/HCA 1995 Annual
Report, 5.
4. Columbia/HCA 1994 Annual
Report, 7.
5. Ibid, 16.
6. Columbia/HCA 1995 Annual
Report, 5.
7. *Business Week,* 18 October
1993; *Wall Street Journal,* 20
January 1994; *Wall Street
Journal,* 12 July 1994.
8. Kevin Lumsdon and Mark
Hagland, "For-Profits—The
Right Medicine for Some
Markets?" *Hospitals and Health
Networks,* 20 June 1994, 34.
9. Mark Hagland, "Eight
Perceptions about For-Profit
Systems," *Hospitals and Health
Networks,* 20 June 1994, 36.
10. *New York Times,* 28 March
1997.
11. Columbia/HCA 1995 Annual
Report, 4–5.
12. Zachary Schiller, Gail
DeGeorge, Stephanie
Anderson Forest, and Eric
Schine, "Balance Sheets That
Get Well Soon," *Business
Week,* 4 September 1995, 81,
84; *Wall Street Journal,* 8 May
1996.
13. Lumsdon and Hagland, "For-
Profits," 41; *Wall Street
Journal,* 9 February 1996;
Wall Street Journal, 30 July
1996.
14. *Wall Street Journal,* 9
September 1996.
15. Kevin Lumsdon, "A Sharper
Edge?" *Hospitals and Health
Networks,* 5 March 1996,
37–38; *Wall Street Journal,* 11
November 1996.

16. Leonard Navarro, "Target Practice," *Hospitals and Health Networks,* 20 December 1996, 16–17.
17. *Wall Street Journal,* 1 May 1996; *Wall Street Journal,* 14 June 1996; *Wall Street Journal,* 21 August 1996, *Wall Street Journal,* 14 March 1997.
18. *Wall Street Journal,* 26 September 1996; Bruce Japsen, "Columbia/HCA Plans $90 Million for Marketing in '97," *Advertising Age,* 17 March 1997, 16; Carey, *Fortunes, Fiddles & Fried Chicken,* 451.
19. Campbell, interview, 12 March 2001.
20. Carey, *Fortunes, Fiddles & Fried Chicken,* 451.
21. Johnson, interview, 9 February 2001.
22. Carey, *Fortunes, Fiddles & Fried Chicken,* 452.
23. Ibid.

Chapter Nine

1. United States Congress, Senate Committee on Governmental Affairs, "Improper Medicare Billing by Hospitals Nationwide for Investigational Devices and Procedures," Washington, D.C.
2. *Wall Street Journal,* 17 July 1997.
3. Lutz and Gee, *Columbia/HCA,* 115–16.
4. Fitzgerald, interview.
5. Lutz and Gee, *Columbia/HCA,* 119–20.
6. *New York Times,* 19 August 1997.
7. Ibid; Kristen Hallem and Deanna Bellandi, "Columbia Probe Has Deep Roots," *Modern Healthcare,* 26 October 1998; Barbara Kirchheimer and Mark Taylor, "$745 Million and Far to Go," *Modern Healthcare,* 22 May 2000, 2.
8. Patricia Sellers, "Don't Mess with Darla," *Fortune,* 8 September 1997, 65; Lutz and Gee, *Columbia/HCA,* 132–33.
9. *Wall Street Journal,* 17 July 1997; *Wall Street Journal,* 25 July 1997.
10. Lutz and Gee, *Columbia/HCA,* 134–35.
11. Sellers, "Don't Mess with Darla," 65; Lutz and Gee, *Columbia/HCA,* 136.
12. New York Times, July 26, 1997; Wall Street Journal, July 28, 1997; Lutz and Gee, *Columbia/HCA,* 136–37.
13. "Corporate Makeover," *Business Nashville,* October 2000, 54.
14. Bob Waterman, interview by the author, tape recording, 9 February 2001, Write Stuff Enterprises.
15. *Wall Street Journal,* 24 March 1997; *Wall Street Journal,* 21 December 1997; *New York Times,* 10 September 1997; Patricia Sellers, "First: The No. 1 Health-Care Company Goes Under the Knife, *Fortune,* 12 January 1998, 27.
16. Bill Choyke, "Ex-HCA Officials Win Their Appeal," *Tennessean,* 25 March 2002; Graham Brink, "Court Clears Ex-HCA executives," *St. Petersburg (Florida) Times,* 26 March 2002.
17. Waterman, interview.
18. *Wall Street Journal,* 15 December 2000.
19. "HCA Announces Understanding to Resolve Remaining Issues in Government Investigation," HCA press release, 18 December 2002.

Chapter Ten

1. "Corporate Makeover," *Business Nashville,* October 2000, 56.
2. Barbara Kirchheimer, "Move Over Columbia, HCA Is Back," *Modern Healthcare,* 19 June 2000.
3. HCA 2000 Annual Report, 4.
4. HCA 1997 Annual Report, 4; *New York Times,* 21 December 1997.
5. "Corporate Makeover," 56–57.
6. HCA 1997 Annual Report, 3–4; HCA 1998 Annual Report, 4; David Rocks, "Columbia/HCA: Showing Signs of Health," *Business Week,* 6 March 6, 2000, 67–68; *Nashville Tennessean,* 25 May 2000.
7. *Nashville Tennessean,* 23 September 1997; *Nashville Banner,* 3 November 1997; *New York Times,* 4 November 1997; *New York Times,* 21 December 1997; *Nashville Tennessean,* 25 May 2000.
8. Bracken, interview, 19 March 2003.
9. Bovender, interview, 8 February 2001.
10. *New York Times,* 25 August 1997; *New York Times,* 21 December 1997; HCA 1997 Annual Report, 4; Michele Bitoun Blecher, "The Redistricting of Columbia," *Hospital and Health Networks,* 20 April 1998, 51; HCA 1999 Annual Report, unpaginated; Rocks, "Columbia/HCA: Showing Signs of Health," 68; *Nashville Tennessean,* 19 March 2000; *Nashville Tennessean,* 5 December 2000.
11. Jack Bovender, interview by the author, recording, 6 March 2003, Write Stuff Enterprises.

12. "Columbia/HCA's Internal Operating Reorganization Plan Signals Return to Local Community Focus," PR Newswire, 17 November 1997.

13. Bracken, interview, 19 March 2003.

14. Barbara Kirchheimer, "Launching the Baby Columbias," *Modern Healthcare*, 3 May 1999, 28; HCA 1998 Annual Report, 2.

15. Barbara Kirchheimer, "Heavyweight Hospitals Build Strength From Within," *Modern Healthcare*, 20 March 2000, 42.

16. HCA 1998 Annual Report, 2.

17. Rocks, "Columbia/HCA: Showing Signs of Health," 68; Kirchheimer, "Heavyweight Hospitals," 43–44; *Nashville Tennessean*, 19 May 2000.

18. HCA 1999 Annual Report.

19. HCA 2001 Annual Report, 5.

20. HCA 1998 Annual Report, 2, 5; HCA 1999 Annual Report.

21. Joe Steakley, interview by the author, recording, 9 February 2001, Write Stuff Enterprises.

22. Rutherford, interview.

23. Information provided by Victor Campbell to Melody Maysonet, May 2003.

24. Information provided by Victor Campbell to Melody Maysonet, 12 December 2001.

25. HCA 2000 Annual Report, 6.

26. Campbell to Maysonet, 14 March 2003.

27. HCA 1999 Annual Report.

28. Campbell to Maysonet, 12 December 2001.

29. Martinez, *Wall Street Journal*, 12 April 2002.

30. Information provided by Jeff Prescott to Melody Maysonet, recording, 2 May 2002.

31. Ibid.

32. Christine Tierney, Kathleen Kerwin, and Charles Haddohenry, "HCA Is Getting Its Strength Back," *Business Week*, 22 April 2002.

33. Prescott to Maysonet, 2 May 2002.

34. Ibid.

35. Milton Johnson, interview by Melody Maysonet, recording, 11 March 2003, Write Stuff Enterprises.

36. Ibid.

37. Information provided by Jim Fitzgerald, June 2003.

38. Johnson, interview, 11 March 2003.

39. Dr. Frank Houser, interview by Melody Maysonet, recording, 14 March 2003, Write Stuff Enterprises.

40. Ibid.

41. Ibid.

42. Ibid.

43. Ibid.

44. Bovender, interview, 6 March 2003.

45. "Thomas Frist Jr., Retiring King of For-profit Health Care," *Nashville Business Journal*, 28 September 2001.

46. Bracken, interview, 9 August 2001.

47. Jack Bovender, interview by the author, recording, 2 February 2001, Write Stuff Enterprises.

48. "HCA's Net Income Decreases 27% Because of Charge," *Wall Street Journal*, 22 October 2002.

49. Bracken, interview, 19 March 2003.

50. Information provided by Sam Hazen, June 2003.

51. Bovender, interview, 6 March 2003.

52. Ibid.

53. Yvette Shields, "Missouri: Sale Gets a Go," *Bond Buyer*, 19 March 2003.

54. HCA 1998 Annual Report, ii.

55. Bracken, interview, 19 March 2003.

56. Ibid.

57. Bovender, interview, 2 February 2001.

**Chapter Ten Sidebar:
Management Team**

1. "Corporate Makeover," *Business Nashville*, October 2000, 56.

**Chapter Ten Sidebar:
Commitment to Communities**

1. "HCA Gives $2 Million to United Way September 11th Fund," PR Newswire, 17 September 2001.

2. "HCA, Labor Department Announce $10 Million Training Program," PR Newswire, 21 December 2001.

3. HCA 2001 Annual Report, 6.

INDEX

Page numbers in italics indicate photographs.